THEY'RE ALL BARKING

A Dog's Guide to Human Behaviour

Professor Daniel Springer-Spaniel F.E.T.C.H.

(Fellow of The European Trust for Canine Health)

Case studies by Doctor Peter Pointer PhD

(Philosopher of Dogs)

They're All Barking

Disclaimer: Please note, Ruth McDonagh is not a veterinarian, dog behaviourist or trainer. The information in this book is intended to raise awareness and act as a guide for dog owners. The author cannot be held responsible for any loss or claim arising out of the use or misuse of suggestions in this book, nor from the failure to take veterinary or other professional advice. Information contained within this book, is correct to the best of Ruth McDonagh's knowledge at the time of publication. Many of the case studies in this book are based on real life incidents. Details of dogs and their owners have been changed. Some examples are fictional, created for literary effect to demonstrate points raised.

First edition independently published in the United Kingdom 2023.

A CIP catalogue record of this book is available from the British Library.

ISBN (Paperback): 978-1-3999720-4-8
ISBN (Hardcover): 978-1-3999753-5-3

Illustrations: Nichola Kingsbury www.NicholaKingsburyart.com
Cover design: Nichola Kingsbury & Matthew J Bird
Typesetting design: Matthew J Bird

For further information about this book, please contact the author at
editor@professordaniel.co.uk

This book is dedicated to dogs everywhere,
in honour of their endless love and devotion to humans.

Contents

Chapter 1

Humans can be quite stupid

The mistake most of my canine comrades make, is thinking that humans are as intelligent as us. They're not. In fact, between you and I, they can be quite stupid.

Unlike us, they've lost the ability to live in the moment and experience sheer joy at the simplest of things. How often do you see your human excitedly – and bare-handedly - digging a deep hole in the garden, their fingers and nails clogged with claggy mud? Rarely. Have you ever seen them running full pelt downstairs with a smelly sock, or pair of dirty pants in their mouths? No, never.

This can be the hardest pill for us canines to swallow - unlike the smelly sock or the lacy pants. Many of you can swallow a cheesy foot-covering, or gulp down a gusset without so much as a by-your-leave – or should I say by-your-heave? We canines naturally exude 'joie de doggie vivre'. Sadly, many of our humans do not. It's the first of many disparities between us and them. If you are to survive in their mad, bad world, you're going to need the steadying reassurance of my guiding paw and the wisdom of my many doggy decades.

Using case studies provided by my esteemed colleague Dr Peter Pointer, PhD (Philosopher of Dogs), I will cite examples in which human behaviour has impacted adversely on a large number of you, causing lasting damage. I'll also quote cases where positive human behaviour has helped mould you into happy, balanced pooches.

Now if I was a gambling professor, I'd stake my box of best beefy biscuits, that some of your humans will want a sneaky peak at this book. If I were you, I'd stash it away so they can't get their sticky fingers on it. I'd suggest you keep it tucked safely under your bed, out of sight. If you rough it up a bit first (your bed not the book), they won't suspect a thing. They'll think you're making a cosy nest. See, I told you they were a bit simple. Everyone knows birds make nests, dogs don't.

It's best to read this book when your humans are out or when they've gone to bed. Be careful not to howl too loudly with laughter or you may wake them. We all know how humans hate being woken in the early hours and forced to traipse downstairs to investigate a strange noise. Should this happen, keep your eyes firmly shut and assume 'deep sleep mode'. Maybe feign a little snore too. This will convince your human that the howling hullabaloo was nothing to do with you. In fact, due to your apparent continued blissful slumber, they'll think there was no noise in the first place. Or, if there was, it was nothing to fear. They'll disappear back to bed, leaving you to resume your rib-tickling read. But, be warned. Whatever you do, don't bury it in the garden. A book does have a spine, but it's not a bone!

Human brains are full of nonsense

I'll be honest with you. Our canine world is a complete mystery to many humans. Most dog-lovers labour under the mistaken belief that we are their pets. While it's true we live in their homes and they feed, walk and care for us, they largely have no idea what we're thinking, or feeling. This makes it very easy to wrap them around our perfectly padded paws.

My research shows that many of you younger canines make the common mistake of thinking humans understand it when you look at them, whine, tilt your head, wag your tail, or run and fetch things for them. A word in your fluffy ears. Human brains are so full of nonsense, they have no room left to receive your messages – no matter how loud and clear you make them. You see the trouble with most humans is they've not learnt our language. Some don't even realise we have a language. Expecting these types of humans to communicate with us is like expecting a goldfish to speak Latin.

For example, how many times do you nudge arms, nose-bump elbows, or scratch their knees to tell them it's time for a walk? The dumber humans probably think you are simply asking for a stroke or a tickle under the chin; the brighter ones may cotton on. In extreme cases, you'll have to fetch your lead and drop it in their lap. Then, with a bit of Lassie luck, your human reaches for their coat and off you both trot – but there's no guarantee.

Similar shenanigans may be required if your belly is rumbling and your human is glued to an inane television programme, or in deep conversation on their mobile. I'm sure you're aware how humans eat as soon as the slightest pang of hunger strikes their oft over-sized stomachs. However, it may be a different starving story for you. You'll learn that human activities often take priority over yours. Once again, it will be down to some persistent pawing on your part, to ensure you're fed at your correct meal-time – and not a minute after.

There may be other situations when you, as the wiser one in the family, will have to protect them. For instance, life-threatening scenarios. These often occur in the middle of the night and will need some sharp action on your part – such as rousing your humans from their deep slumber. They'll be dreaming of holidays in the sun or longed for unattainable loves, unaware of the smoky dangers lurking in their lounge, or some shifty ne'er-do-well who's about to jemmy open the dining room window and make off with some of your family's beloved 'stuff'.*

If you've barked or whined yourself hoarse to no avail, you'll be forced to pull at pillows, nip at nighties and disrupt duvets, to alert them to the smouldering sofa or unwelcome intruder. Once they're awake, prepare for panic-stricken action stations with emergency calls, donning of dressing gowns and safe fleeing of said smouldering or violated home. If you're lucky, your human will remember to take you with them!

*Stuff: Something else you will learn when living with a human. A lot of them tend to enjoy accumulating stuff. Some of it simply adorns their homes and gardens and has no practical value. The old adage, 'it's neither use nor ornament,' is quite apt. These stuff-gathering humans could learn a thing or two from you. You've a cosy bed (hopefully), a water bowl, a feeding bowl, a collar and lead and perhaps a few toys and treats. That's your lot in life – and I expect that 99 per cent of the time you are much happier and enjoying each day far more than your hoarding human.

What you must always keep at the forefront of your doggy mind is that humans are simply not like you. You can spend your lifetime trying to communicate with them, but whether you succeed is another matter - and definitely not down to any lack of effort on your part.

Dr Peter Pointer gives this analogy.
Imagine you are Human 1.

"There are two humans talking on their mobiles. Human 1 is on top of a cliff, while Human 2 is standing at the foot of the cliff with intermittent reception. The signal from Human 1's mobile goes out loud and clear, but Human 2's phone receives only crackly and stilted information. Instead of moving from below the cliff, Human 2 becomes frustrated, waving their arms about, tripping over a stone as they walk backwards and forwards. They eventually give up and turn off the mobile.

"The same communication mismatch happens frequently between a canine and its human. A dog's signals are transmitted loudly and clearly, but are not always received, for a whole variety of reasons."

"To get a clearer signal, Human 2 should move away from the cliff for a better reception, climbing up steps if necessary. The result would be effective two-way communication and understanding. Unfortunately, Human 2 (representative of many dog-owners) either a) Doesn't wish to make the physical effort of climbing steps or b) The thought doesn't enter their head. Instead, they remain doggedly (ironically) at the foot of the metaphorical cliff – and your signals are never picked up."

Now I believe one of the reasons that many humans don't find the time to communicate with you is due to what I call their head haze. The more time you spend with humans (and yes, I've spent a lot), you will learn that they harbour thoughts only two-legged beings could conjure up. For instance: What colour should I paint my nails? Did I renew my gym membership? Do these shoes go with this coat? What tattoo should I have? When did we last clean out the fridge? Did you remember to put out the rubbish? Shall we get more of those nice chocolate biscuits? Which film shall we watch tonight? When is my hairdresser's appointment? Did you download that new shopping app?

We canines have no time or need for these humdrum conundrums. For us, there are far more real and important matters to enjoy: Digging a hole, (see earlier), swallowing a sock (see earlier), gnawing that new bone, exploring a mouse hole, chasing a rabbit or bird, snapping at flies, or snoozing in the sun.

Humans put high importance on the unimportant

You will discover that humans put high importance on the most unimportant things. Things to which we canines would never give a second sniff. Things that in the grand scheme of life, carry very little weight.

For example, we never paint our nails – and may Doggie Heaven preserve us if any human thinks that's a good idea! We don't routinely require shoes – unless of course you've a delicate paw issue. Some of our racing colleagues do have ear tattoos, but this is not by choice. If we had a fridge, obviously we'd lick it clean daily. Rubbish is to be sniffed, pawed at and eaten, and ditto for biscuits - though not chocolate ones. To snuffle those could mean a painful stomach and a trip to the vet, as I know some of you have found out.

I concede that some of us do find certain human films of interest. Wildlife documentaries and animal programmes are particularly entertaining. Seeing deer, squirrels or rabbits race across your living room or hearing birds squawking or sheep bleating, is enough to whet any healthy hound's appetite. Your human will find it highly amusing (or annoying) that you take such a keen interest. But avidly watching wildlife and barking whilst attempting to hunt down your prey as it disappears behind the telly, are your natural instincts. Don't let their reactions make you feel like you're the mad one. As you'll soon learn, in truth, it is they who are the mad ones.

I know some of you endure regular trips to the hairdresser - in doggy parlance the groomer. When I was a pup, groomers didn't exist. I know some of you grow very thick, long or curly coats. If left untrimmed for too many moons, then yes, you'll get matted, tangled and suffer great discomfort. In these cases, I agree that some preventative, or even remedial trimming and cutting is required. But by and large, what I term this 'airy-fairy frippery' appeals more to image-conscious humans than it does to us dogs.

Humans do seem to enjoy frequenting these pong-filled parlours with their wallets wide open. Some seem to go whether the dog needs it or not. These humans prefer their pets smelling like - and please excuse my 'chien francais' - a bitch's boudoir. In some cases, they look not dissimilar to said bitch themselves. Think silky bows, studded collars, blow-dried curls and even – may GOD DOG save us - coloured tints.

Call me old-fashioned, but let me warn you, you'll be chained up like a canine gimp and forcibly man or woman-handled – and that is no canine's idea of fun. I do feel for those of you who have to undergo this type of restraint and re-styling on a regular basis. You're soaked, shampooed and expected to stand still to be dried with a thunderous blower of rocket-proportions. For dog salon, think canine house of horrors. Unsurprisingly, I know it proves too much for some of you. I've heard of many a hound becoming a quivering wreck during these grooms and others whose nerves have been blow-dried to oblivion by well-meaning humans.

What humans think are 'good ideas' often aren't

As we all know, any self-respecting and balanced canine is its own dog. We have our own thoughts and emotions, our own wishes and desires. By and large, they don't involve salons, blow-dries, dyes and tints, colourful outdoor clothes, silky ribbons, or other hair-brained human accessories. What some humans believe are good ideas, we canines know unequivocally, are not.

In the following chapters, I will take you through some of the common pitfalls of being an 'owned pet.' I'll explain the types of humans with whom you may share your life and their pros and cons. Some are great, some not so great; some are simply thoughtless and some just simple. Others – and thankfully this is the minority – are downright cruel.

I'll explain the differences you can expect in human and canine communication and how understanding and misunderstanding are so easily confused.

You may be one of those dogs who believes life is best approached at 120 mph. If you've not been advised or taught otherwise, your exuberance for life will soon wear thin with your humans. You'll find that whatever you do, you can't put a

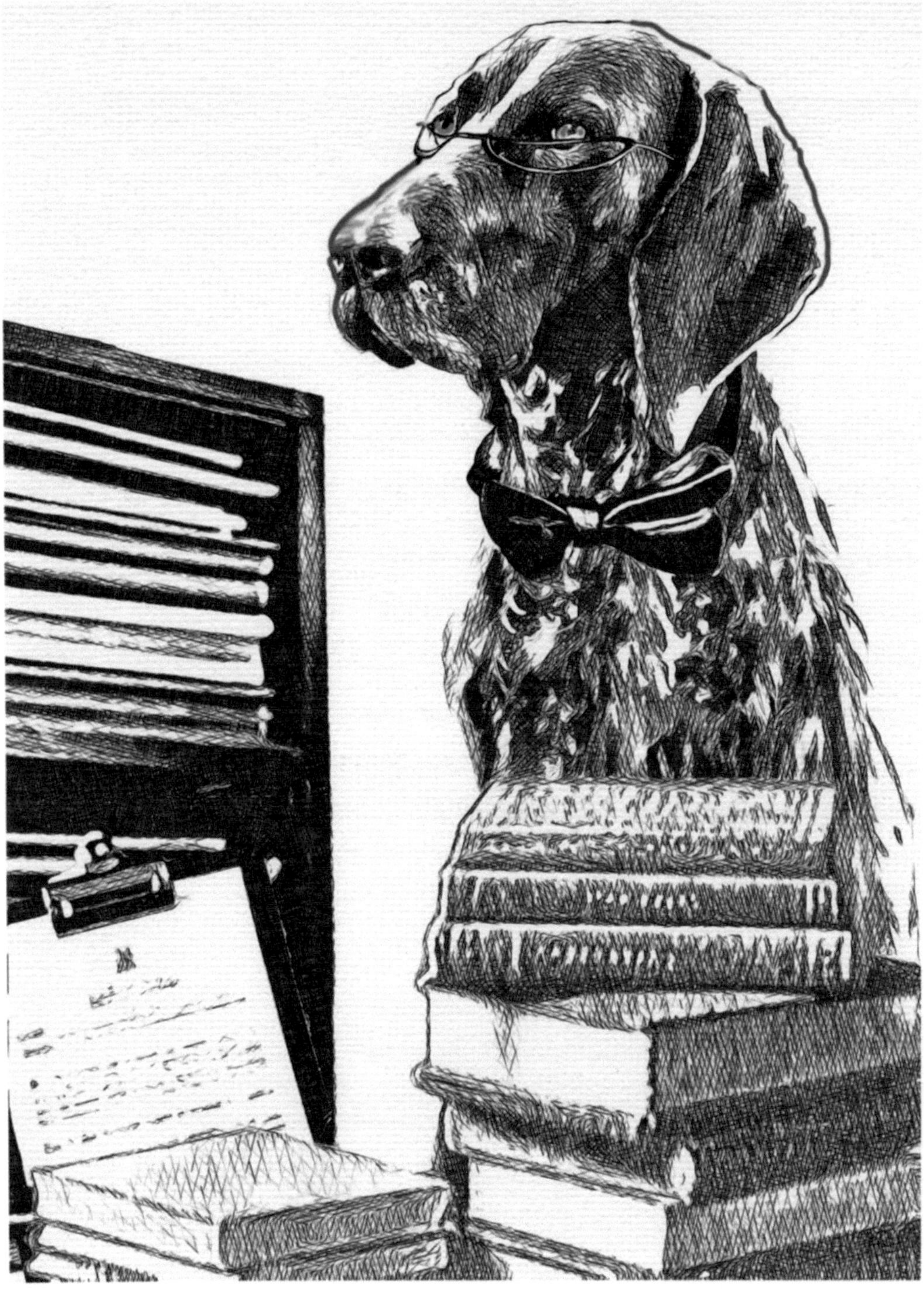

"I'm using case studies provided by my esteemed colleague, Dr Peter Pointer PhD (Philosopher of Dogs)."

paw right. As a lovable, cuddly pup you were the apple of their eye. But 12 months on, you're seen only as a bad apple. You'll receive nothing but scoldings and little positive encouragement. Without appropriate human behaviour – and I must be honest, there is a lot of inappropriate human behaviour out there - you'll discover how your life can turn from being all hunky doggy to pitifully sad and sorry.

I hope that by reading this guide to human behaviour you will be better-equipped to cope with the ups and downs of living with these strange two-legged creatures. With this behavioural awareness in your canine memory cupboard alongside some practised inner resilience, you may stand a fighting chance of coming out the other end of the experience slightly less scathed.

Professor Daniel's Bones of Retention:

- **Humans can be quite stupid**
- **They dwell on unimportant matters**
- **Humans live in the past or the future**
- **Our communication signals go over their heads (or through their legs)**
- **Beware of humans with 'good ideas'**
- **Keep this book well-hidden (but don't bury it in the garden)**
- ***You* are not the mad one**

Chapter 2

You're not 'just a dog'

If you ever overhear anyone referring to you as just a dog, I strongly recommend you pee up their leg. Initially, your human mum or dad will be mortified. They class weeing on a person as embarrassing and disrespectful. But take it from me, any human worth their salt will be secretly impressed that you put such an ignoramus in their rightful, urine-soaked place. In fact, they will probably have a good giggle once the wet-legged lummox is out of earshot.

Just a dog indeed! But this is an attitude you may face from unenlightened humans who don't realise just how wonderful you are. I could refer to these sorts of ignorant people as 'just humans'.

Now some humans will think mistakenly, that buying and owning a pet will be all sweetness and light. Beware these humans, for they tend to live in a fantasy doggy dreamland where everything is fluffy, furry, cuddly and curly. After collecting you from a breeder or rescue centre, they anticipate you trotting home with them, not a care in the world and living happily ever after.

They imagine you will sit in a corner, quietly accepting fuss and doing as you're told. Of course, I love a head rub, ear massage or belly scratch as much as the next dog (especially those that make your back leg go scratch, scratch, scratch, thump, thump, thump). But we canines are so much more than that. Be warned. Some people do not know this (because they are just humans) and it can make for an uncomfortable and even unhappy partnership.

Humans make inane comments

A large number of humans, even the brighter ones, don't appreciate our intelligence and sensitivity. As mentioned earlier, some of you go to extreme lengths and place yourselves in harm's way to warn and save your humans from life-threatening situations. Even with such clear evidence in front of their rosy, smooth faces, you will hear these humans and their family and friends making the most inane and uninformed comments.

For example: "Do you think the dog knew you were in danger?"

"I can't believe a dog could do that!"

"That's amazing, he must have known..."

These incredulous statements serve only to support my theory that some humans don't have the slightest idea how clever and knowing you are.

If further proof is needed, look at our much-admired and respected canine colleagues who work within the police, fire, search and rescue and medical assistance fields. I appreciate a lot of these canines are at the top of their doggy games. These exceptional individuals are singled out at an early age for their insight and intelligence. They spend months or even years training in their specialist area, some even being awarded the highest honours for their courage and life-saving skills.

Sniffing it out – your exceptional snout

Admittedly, not all of us are leading scent-trackers, drug-sniffers, finders of missing persons, or able to warn of a human seizure. But we all have, in varying degrees, natural instincts and intelligence. You all have those same impressive qualities within you, but your humans often don't realise it – maybe because many of them have lost the ability to tap into their own.

One of your outstanding talents is of course your sense of smell. Thankfully, humans do know that our noses are much more efficient and useful than theirs. From what I've seen, humans use theirs only for sneezing, snoring, snorting illegal substances, sniffing flowers, food and wine, or poking them into other people's business. I've yet to see a human sniff out the seat of a fire, track the path of a lost hill walker, or uncover truffles.

Some humans do use their noses in their work, such as perfumiers and sommeliers, but very few compared to us. Human noses are simply fleshy, holey appendages that humans enjoy picking, especially when in their cars or watching the telly. They complain about some of our habits, but I've never seen a canine with a claw up his snout.

Our superior abilities don't stop at scenting. Many of our natural senses are better than theirs, including, in many cases, common sense.

The human nose contains a paltry five million olfactory receptors...I know, I'm howling with laughter too. (For the pups among you, the Olfactory Cortex is the part of the brain concerned with the sense of smell.) The human's miniscule five million receptors are like a flea in a field compared with the 300 million we canines possess. As we all know, this means our sense of smell is between 10,000 and 100,000 times more sensitive than theirs and 10,000 times more accurate. We also devote around 30 per cent of our brains to detecting and identifying odours, whereas humans use only 5 per cent of theirs. No whiff of a surprise there.

How often have your tried to tell your human their toast is burning, that there's a fox skulking in the garden, the neighbour's cat is pooing on the gravel, or there's a hedgehog hibernating in a pile of leaves? Nine times out of ten, you'll be told in no uncertain terms to be quiet and go away.

When humans don't understand our communications, they'll assume you are making an unnecessary fuss. They'll dismiss your attempt to attract their attention with a 'stop being silly', or 'go and lie down'. If they could tear themselves away from whatever important mobile app they are viewing and connect with you for a moment, they may have a fighting chance of understanding your messages. Perhaps if your face appeared on a mobile app, you would be more likely to get their attention.

Your nifty nose tells you everything

What they also don't realise is that your nifty nose means they can't keep any secrets from you. You always know who's been in their house, even if you're not there at the time.

You may return home from a lovely walk to find Grandma's heavily perfumed aroma still hanging around the house, hours after her departure. You'll take in the sweaty whiff of a long-gone footballing teenager who was on a ravenous foray to the fridge. If the neighbour's cat has visited the hamster - you'll know that too. Should the supermarket delivery driver spill the shopping, you'll know at which exact spot and rush to help clean it up.

If your human has given some 'unknown' a lift in the car, you'll know that too. Whether it be animal, vegetable, mineral or other, you can sniff it out before your human can say "Achoo".

I'm sure some humans are jolly glad you can't talk – for many a sordid tale you could tell. I know some of you have been privy to your mum or dad's secret visitors when they were home alone. In such circumstances they think your presence doesn't count. What they don't appreciate - because they are just humans (and there are no humans as stupid as those in love or lust), is that you take it all in. You know exactly what's going on. If you find yourself witnessing such domestic skulduggery, I suggest giving your errant human 'the look'. By that I mean to wear your most serious face. Follow them around (including upstairs if you're allowed), but do not under any circumstance, entertain any tail-wagging. Keep a discreet but disapproving distance.

It's likely your human will be so distracted by their secret guest that they will be oblivious to your furry frowns. But if they do notice your disapproving doggie demeanour, they may suffer some guilt pangs. I can guarantee this will result in the door being slammed on your sensitive snout. I'd suggest retiring to your bed and not emerging until the rest of the family are home. It's likely your human will seek you out once their guest has gone, keen to make amends. If you give their guilt-laden advances a subdued shun and lie low, they may get your message and you might even get a biscuit out of it.

Humans love so-called 'nice smells'

One odd obsession a lot of humans have, is wearing pungent aftershave or strong perfume. In this situation, your sensitive snouts are likely to be more of a hindrance than a help. You'll find these two-legged chemical carriers do literally get up your nose. Many humans love to squirt and splash, very liberally. They adore these so-called nice smells. It's about making themselves feel more appealing, acceptable or even attractive to others. Sometimes it's to help attract a partner or mate, to impress people generally, for their own pleasure or to mask their body smells. However, unless you can escape these sinus-inflaming aromas, be warned - they can give you a hounding headache.

NB: Wearing artificial smells isn't something you'll ever need to do. You're attracted to (or repelled from) mates or friends after a good bottom inhalation. There is so much information you can glean from a quick – or long – bum sniff. Coupled with body language, you can tell immediately if you've met this particular dog before, if they are male or female, their general health, mood and diet.

It's not something a lot of humans do as they don't have the scent sense, or the easy bottom access like you do. (Some humans may, but that's not appropriate content for this book.)

Beware their air freshening obsessions

On the subject of pungent pongs, be warned that many humans are also obsessed with aerosol air fresheners and plug-in room scenters. They hate and fear the thought of your pongy doggy smell in their homes – especially if you're wet. In the winter, after a muddy, rainy walk, you return home, the windows are closed, the heating is on and your human resorts to these so-called air fresheners to keep their rooms smelling sweet.

It's possible some of these plug-in room fresheners may contain VOCs – volatile organic compounds. These VOCs cause any chemicals in the device to vaporise at room temperature, releasing said nice smell. As with most chemicals, they are potentially hazardous to both you and your human, especially if you already have any type of breathing issues.

Humans tend to place these plug-in appliances right at your sniffing level. They will 'pissssh pisssh' in your face at random times of the day and night. If they catch you unawares, they'll give you an unwelcome blast of sickly sweetness. If the room has no natural ventilation, it's likely to be become a pretty perfume-laden, less-than-perfect environment for you.

You may have seen those scent sticks that stand proudly perfumed in a glass jar on the side. Give those a wide berth too. Your human has access to all kinds of these artificial room scenters, but the most unpleasant ones, as far as you're concerned, are usually manufactured in some far-flung Asian factory and sold cheaply. They contain all types of strong chemicals and will do you no good at all.

Oils aren't always essential

Humans with a few more pennies in their pockets, may opt for the natural essential oil room scenters. Generally, these are better quality and more expensive, but even some natural oils can make you poorly. They could potentially irritate your respiratory system if you are exposed to them for long periods.

Were you to ingest some after a spill, or should it get rubbed on your skin, or absorbed through your fur, it could prove fatal. You should be particularly wary of concentrated forms of clove oil, citrus oil, pine oil, peppermint oil, oil of wintergreen, cinnamon oil, eucalyptus oil and tea tree oil.

Essential oils are of course used regularly by professionals who apply zoopharmacognosy to animals. Yes, that's a very long word but I am a Professor after all! It refers to when animals self-select plants, herbs, oils or minerals to help heal themselves. (A bit like when you eat grass to help your digestion.) The difference with this is that *you* select, often by sniffing, what you need.

In your human home you probably have little choice but to inhale whatever scent – pure or potentially harmful – is in the air. If you do find any scents sickening and you're able to move elsewhere, getting your sensitive snout out of harm's way, may be a good idea.

Personally, chemical scents make me feel sick. Tox-sick in fact. If I had my way, they'd all be 'scent' packing. Our feline friends are particularly susceptible to essential oils. I've heard of some nearly losing one of their nine lives after accidently inhaling these substances. Even felines wouldn't be so stupid as to deliberately inhale toxic substances.

If your human had our powerful scenting skills and crawled about on all fours with their noses to the ground as we do, they might rethink some of their household habits.

Case study: Larry the Lurcher

Larry's mum bought a plug-in tea tree oil diffuser for her lounge. Little did she know how it would affect her beloved pet. Larry tells Dr Peter Pointer what he remembers of that fateful day.

"It was a normal day. I'd had a nice walk and my breakfast and Mum went off to work. I stretched out on the sofa and drifted off to sleep. When I woke up later, I felt most strange. There was a pungent smell in the room and my nose and throat were sore and inflamed. I got up for a drink of water and I felt all wobbly. My legs didn't want to work properly and I was very cold. I flopped down on the floor and went back to sleep. The next I knew was a woman was waking me up. I felt very scared as I didn't recognise her. (Apparently it was Mum.) I couldn't stand up and felt very disoriented, so I crawled under a chair. I was drooling and couldn't stop shaking. When I came to, I was at the vets. There were needles and things under my skin and I think I was on a drip. Whatever it was, I was feeling better. Once I was allowed home, I heard Mum saying it was her new oil diffuser that had poisoned me. She said we were lucky it hadn't damaged my liver. Mum threw the smelly thing away and never bought another."

Mind your paws on bleachy floors

Bleach-laden floor cleaners are another pet hate of mine. Some cleaning fluids that humans happily slosh around, are a chemical cocktail of corrosive nasties as far as you're concerned. Many owners don't realise that if you walk across a recently-washed floor, you can end up with bleachy feet and absorb these unhealthy horrors through your paws. Many humans are blissfully unaware of this and mop away merrily, keen on killing 99.9% of germs without realising the potential short, or long-term effect on you. Keep well away if you can and don't under any circumstances, lick your paws afterwards. It's best not to ingest sodium hypochlorite.

Exceptional ears – your superpower

Hearing, is of course your other outstanding sense. As with your scenting, this is a well-known doggy fact that many humans DO know. But they don't always consider how it can affect you in your everyday life. Able to detect sounds up to a mile away, your eminent ears receive loud and clear vibrations of up to 50,000 Hertz per second – compared with humans who are stuck at a lowly 20,000 Hertz. (Again, for the youngsters among you, Hertz is a measure of sound frequency and the higher the frequency, the higher the pitch of the sound.) You can hear high-pitched noises so you can hunt down squeaky mice and other prey that may squeal, scream or scurry. When you lived in the wild, it was also an early-warning system for potential foe, aiding your survival.

Though a great asset to your early ancestors, when tucked up with your humans in cosy domesticity, it can be a challenging aural cross you have to bear. Your cloth-eared human will think nothing of turning up the volume on a sound system to near deafening proportions as you snooze on the sofa.

Bellowing at the telly during some ball game is another favourite of theirs. You are transported from happily napping to near heart-failure in seconds. They're also good at starting up the chainsaw, hedge trimmer, or lawnmower just a few feet from your half-pricked ears as you dreamily soak up the summer sun. Power drilling above your bed is another favourite. These thoughtless DIY doggie deafeners will cause you to flee scared, ears ringing and nerves frazzled to escape their unbearable, electric frenzy.

Humans do hear these sounds, but at a much lower volume than us – hence their insensitivity. They have no idea of the intense ear-bashing their weekend pastimes can bestow upon us. You would probably have to sit in a corner with your paws over your ears for your human to realise how uncomfortable and sometimes even frightening such loud domestic noises can be. In the wireless fidelity age in which we're now all living, your home is also bombarded with constant high-frequency sounds and waves of which your human is likely to be blissfully unaware.

Humans love fireworks of explosive magnitude

Talking of noise, another unpleasant habit humans have, is letting off very loud fireworks. This often happens around Guy Fawkes night and New Year's Eve. There will likely be other random nights of nauseous noise too, as and when they celebrate individual birthdays, anniversaries and other such human hurrahs.

I know this bizarre behaviour sends thousands of you running scared, with many more left quaking, shaking, drooling and panting. The sheer ferocity and volume of this man-made madness has to be seen and unfortunately heard, to be believed.

When I was a pup, humans were happy with pretty sparklers and the odd Catherine Wheel or glittery rocket, whose bang though scary, we could just about handle. Be on your guard. In this commercially-driven age, humans vie to outdo each other by buying the biggest, best, brightest, loudest and most expensive of everything. Fireworks are no exception. Many humans will seek out the loudest, noisiest explosives they can find.

Sadly, those who bear the brunt are us canines and any furry friends who live with you, as well as farmed and wild animals. I've heard of sheep having heart attacks in fields, literally being frightened to death by these ferocious fireworks filling the night sky. I've heard of horses bolting in fright, ripping themselves asunder on barbed wire. Roosting birds can be so petrified they fall from trees with heart failure. It does us and all these other sensitive souls no good whatsoever to be subjected to such celebratory events.

If you have a considerate human, they'll do all they can to avoid you being within earshot of these horrific explosions. Some humans may give you calming medication, other may put you in, or under, a comforting blanket. I know some of you will be taken away from any explosive-filled areas altogether. I find fireworks one of the many unfathomable foibles of the human world. To me, it's inexplicably selfish and it's something we canines (and other animal friends) have to endure, often in fear and aural agony.

Case study: Bustle the Jack Russell

Like many Jack Russell Terriers, Bustle is an intelligent little chap. When his mum Sue, was invited to a firework party at a friend's house, she took Bustle along too. Bustle recalls the fateful night to Dr Peter Pointer:

"I could sense Mum was looking forward to something, because she was talking to me in an excitable way as she put on my winter coat. Mum was happy so I was happy, I thought maybe we were having a wintry evening walk in the moonlight, full of sniffs. How wrong I was. We turned up at her friend's house in the country where a big bonfire was blazing in a nearby field. I noticed there were no other dogs around. I kept close to Mum's legs as I sensed something was going to happen. Mum was laughing and smiling and drinking something that smelled strong. All of a sudden, this massive whizz, flash and bang came out of nowhere. It petrified me. I lay glued to the ground but my whole body was shaking, I tried to hide behind Mum's legs, but couldn't escape the noise. She didn't seem to notice. She was busy looking into the sky and saying "ooh". This horrendous ordeal went on for what seemed like ages. The noise was incredibly loud and the flashing so bright. Mum picked me up which helped a bit, but it didn't stop the noise. When we got home, I hid under the sofa and wouldn't come out all night. I felt sick and exhausted and my ears were ringing. For the rest of the week, I didn't want to go out of the house. Now I'm too scared to go for a walk in the dark which seems to annoy Mum. If I hear cars back-firing or doors banging, I start shaking. I never used to feel nervous but now I'm scared of any sudden, or loud noises. Mum says I'm being silly and has taken me to the vet to talk about

sedatives. I was quite happy until we went to that bonfire. It terrified me."

Hooray for low noise fireworks!

But there is light on the horizon – and it's not of the dazzling, cracking, ear-splitting, eye-blinding variety. Quieter, more dog-friendly fireworks are now available and are being used by some caring humans. These pretty but more peaceful explosives are making their midnight mark thanks to animal-loving campaigners. These considerate humans appreciate the deep distress the unspeakably loud and thunderous fireworks cause us (and other creatures). The arrival of low-noise, or animal- friendly options is excellent news for all animals of whatever persuasion. It's a reassuring sign that some humans do sympathise with how sensitive our natures are.

Talking of thunder, I know tumultuous storms and gales are just as frightening for some of you, along with back-firing cars and gunshots. If your human is unaware of this, prepare for bouts of anxiety-inducing ear-bashings from which there's little escape. It's no wonder some of you have to hide under your human's bed, or cower terrified in the corner.

Again, your human may gently scold you for being silly, telling you there's nothing to fear. Now we know that 'being silly' doesn't come into it. It's physically uncomfortable and frightening for you, but getting this message across to your human is not easy. If you stood them blindfolded behind a jet engine before take-off, maybe they would understand and be more sympathetic.

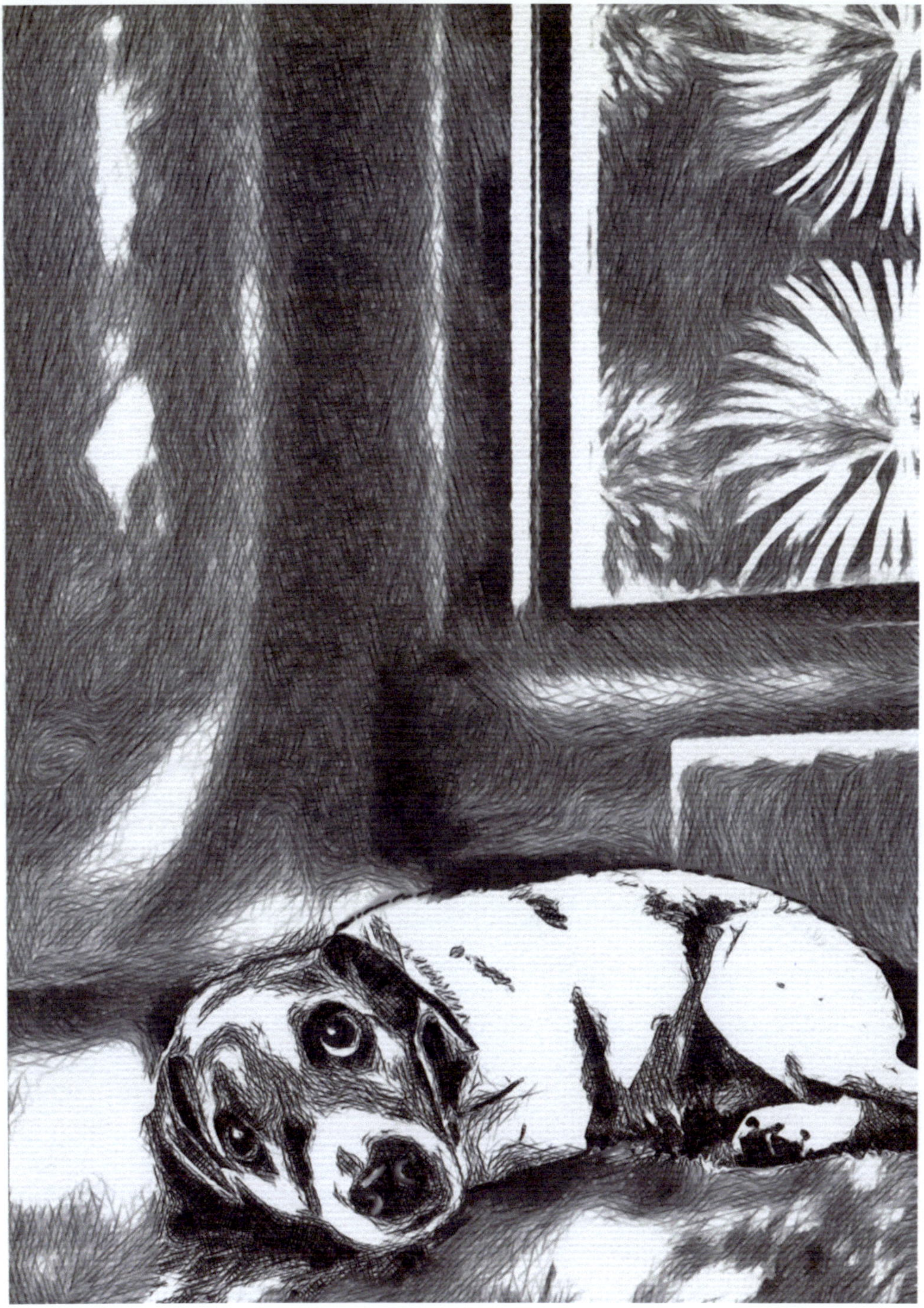

"Fireworks are of explosive magnitude and leave thousands of you quaking, shaking, drooling and panting."

Professor Daniel's Bones of Retention:

- Wee on a human who says you're just a dog
- You have superpower senses
- Humans can't sniff their way out of a paper bag
- Avoid harmful chemicals
- Humans are cloth-eared
- You are not 'silly'
- Low-noise fireworks are our new best friend

Chapter 3

Sensing your human's emotions

Your ability to simply 'sense' your human's emotions is another doggie quality your human may have great difficulty in understanding or appreciating. Be careful. This is one of the biggest threats to your health and well-being when sharing your life with humans.

Many of them don't realise that you absorb their stress and anxiety and sometimes even their physical pain and tension. In fact, you may feel it just as acutely, if not more so, than them. Merely living in a hectic household day after day, is very damaging for you. What many humans don't know is that, much like the high-pitched sound waves, their feelings carry a vibration, to which you are highly sensitive.

A lot of humans can't see or hear these themselves, so it makes it hard, if not impossible for the majority of them to grasp the concept. For many humans, if they can't see it, feel it, smell it or hear it, it doesn't exist – though of course we know different.

As you're much more in touch with your natural senses than most humans, you instinctively pick up and feel these vibrations. Some humans call it energy. Just like hearing and sniffing, it's one of our intuitive senses. Humans have it too, but it's dormant in many.

Look out for the following common, human experiences that could affect you and for which you should be prepared with your best paws forward. These include:

Losing a human in your household

Losing a human through a bereavement or a relationship break-up, are both heart-breaking and emotionally-charged experiences for you and your human. We feel loss as much as the next being – human or animal – and we grieve. The good news is you're likely to move on more quickly than your human. In that instance, you'll need to be patient and loving, to help get your human through what may be a dark time for them. It's vital you show them their life is worth living and there is still love and light in the world, in other words, you're there.

Getting them up in the morning, preparing your breakfast, taking you out for walks and meeting other dog-owners, will help get them through. Getting out in nature and socialising is an important release for you too. You will absorb their grief, but you also need to release it.

Living with highly-stressed humans

This is a very regular occurrence in the 21st century and one I see all too frequently. A stressed human usually means a stressed dog. You'd have to be a canine with a heart of concrete (and I don't think such a thing exists) not to be adversely impacted by your owner's stress. Being loving, loyal companions, your job is again, to support and care for your human. But this means it's nigh on impossible for you not to soak up their emotions, giving you unwelcome levels of anxiety and angst that are not of your making. Enjoying lots of walks, a nice doggie massage, scent games, swimming and playing with friends, can all help release your emotional tension.

Case study: Tiger the Yorkshire Terrier

Tiger is like a pea on a drum. He sleeps with one ear open and rushes around the house if anyone comes in. He regularly stands at the window barking at passing dogs and people. Here he tells Dr Peter Pointer why:

"My mum is a busy woman and rarely sits down and relaxes. She is always on the go and always has something to do. She talks quickly into her phone and taps nearly as quickly on her laptop. This is when she isn't exercising. Our house is always a whirl of activity. I have to keep pace with it or I may miss out. Mum doesn't relax so I don't feel I can either. I need to be on my guard, ready to get up and go, just like Mum. When she's talking loudly on her phone I keep watch, shouting at other dogs to keep away if I see them outside. It's quite an exhausting life, but I love my mum to bits and as she never stops, neither do I."

Living with anxious or depressed humans

These emotions create another type of negative, dense environment for you and there's a fear you may end up being dragged down to their despairing level. Of course, as their canine, your role is to love, support and care for your human – whatever feelings befall them. It is extremely sad when you know your human is void of any emotional vibrance and again, your job is to provide them with stability and love.

Showing them that life can be a more joyful experience is something you can do through simple acts of doggy kindness. Licking their hands or face, nuzzling them warmly when they're feeling particularly low or crying, taking them their shoes or slippers, drawing their attention to the outside world. You need to encourage them to take you out for a walk and much of the advice I've given for the first two scenarios, will also apply to you here.

Living with an angry or violent human

These individuals create a highly-charged, negative environment and one that could create a physical risk to you. It's most unfortunate if you're doomed to share this type of home. There is no doubt it will drain and deject you, maybe even leading to depression.

Due to your love and loyalty, you find it exceptionally hard to protect yourself emotionally, from situations like this. In extreme cases, where physical or emotional violence is involved, putting up a barrier against your human is the only way you will survive.

I'm aware of some canines who end up completely shutting down, that is to say turning in on themselves emotionally. These poor, unfortunate souls have endured such negativity and abuse, they can no longer show any emotion. They are so overwhelmed by fear and disappointment, they can only sit, head hanging and hunched, unable to respond to any human interaction. Others, whose spirits aren't quite broken, will turn to violence themselves, becoming aggressive, snarling and biting. This is merely an act of self-preservation, a last resort and final attempt to reclaim some control over their sad, sorry lives.

Case study: Steffie the rescue Staffie

Fiona was going through a difficult time at work and in her personal life. She thought rehoming a rescue dog would get her outdoors and help her relax. She re-homed Steffie, a boisterous young Staffie, with an unknown history. She told Dr Peter Pointer how it ended in yet more tears.

"When I first met Fiona, I could tell she was a very unhappy woman. She had a sad aura about her. She liked my exuberant nature and decided to adopt me. She'd bought me a lovely comfy bed, a smart collar and lead and all sorts of amazing squeaky toys. I felt very lucky to have arrived in such a great home. But as the weeks went by, Fiona's attitude towards me changed. The novelty of having me in her life began to wear off. I wasn't the dog she expected me to be and her already high level of stress began to affect me. I'd never lived full-time in a house, so I'd not learnt to do my business outside. I found it hard to hold on overnight and if I made a mess, Fiona was very cross with me in the morning. She would raise her voice and bang about. All I did was sit and shake. When we went out for walks, I got very excited. I loved meeting other dogs and people. She'd complain that I didn't do as I was told and that I was too strong for her. She scolded me for not coming back and for pulling her around. Sometimes she would lose her temper and shout at me. That upset me even more and I'd wee where I stood. My walks got shorter and less frequent; some days I didn't go out at all. I rarely saw any other people or dogs and that made me sadder. There was no one to have fun with.

Fiona would get very irritated when I squeaked my toys. She didn't like me chewing them as I left bits on the floor. Some evenings she would shout at me because I was making too much noise. I'd cower in a corner, not really sure what I'd done, but I knew she didn't want me there. Then she'd start crying. I hated it when she cried and I felt like crying too. I wanted to lick her hand and nuzzle up to her, but I was scared of being scolded, so I stayed in my bed. I felt very miserable. I heard her on the phone to a friend one night. She said I was making her more stressed and wasn't fitting into her life as she'd hoped. She was thinking of taking me back to the rescue centre. I felt very anxious and my tummy began churning. That night, I made an awful smelly mess in the kitchen. I didn't do it on purpose, but felt very stressed myself. Later that day we went on a car journey. The staff at the rescue centre made a big fuss of me. Fiona gave them my comfy bed and squeaky toys. I spent all evening playing with them and no one told me off."

Sensing and sharing in a human's joy

While you sense your human's negative emotions, the good news is, you also react to their positive ones too. They may be ones of excitement, happiness, anticipation or joy. (Yes, they do feel it sometimes.)

Maybe they've come home with a new toy or a special treat for you. You'll immediately know from their tone of voice and demeanour that something exciting is about to happen. Perhaps someone in the human family has achieved success at school, received a promotion at work, secured a new job or come first in a sports competition.

This creates an upbeat aura of happiness. Warmth and smiles will fill your home (and you'll probably also get a few special cuddles into the bargain). Humans love to share their happiness with you and though you may not know exactly what's gone on, you'll have a pretty good idea. You will love nothing more than joining in with the happy feeling by padding around wagging your tail and licking anyone in your path and receiving fuss in return.

A joyful human means a joyful dog

In my experience, it's less common for humans to experience (unlike you), the feeling of sheer joy. This usually surfaces only at times of important events during human lives such as births, engagements, weddings, family reunions, or major achievements.

Now, oddly enough, this is also where you come in. Your human may not realise this, but if they were to work or train with you, the feeling they would get when you accomplish things together as a team, is indeed that of sheer joy. And of course, as your human's team-mate, what they feel, you'll feel, so it's a big beefy win for you too. A joyful human creates a joyful dog.

Your human may take you to training classes such as agility, scenting or trailing. Collies may find themselves in sheep dog trials or fly-ball competitions, while any manner of dog may be found walking proudly around a dog show ring. Any achievement by you (that admittedly they've probably had a small hand in) will bring them great pleasure. They won't know it until it happens, particularly if they've never involved you in such things before. It's a fantastic canine-human experience that they – and you - are clearly missing out on. They will have no idea what bliss you can bring them.

Working together to achieve a shared goal – whether there's a prize at the end or not – can bring them that rare human feeling of utter joy. Of course, you'll share in that too, in your own doggy way. There may be some bouncing, happy barking, molar-filled laughter, circling, jumping, running or zoomies. It matters not how you show your delight, the important thing is that you and your human share it. A joint accomplishment achieved together, is a wonderful experience for you and for them.

Creating a calm connection

Now a less exuberant emotion I sincerely hope you get to experience, is that of calm connection with your human. As I've said in earlier chapters, many humans do live busy, hectic, stress-filled lives, with much coming, going, to-ing and fro-ing and with little down time. You may find yourself being slotted in, as and when your human can manage. This type of household is one where calm connection would do everyone, human and dog alike the peaceful, power of good.

The chances of your human being disconnected from you, are probably far higher, than them actually being connected to you. Don't get me wrong, some humans are in tune with us – and do feel for us and other living beings. But a word of caution, many are not.

If your humans regularly take time out to be calm, they can connect not only with you, but with nature in general. Like you, humans need to just sit and be, thinking not of tomorrow or next week, but of now, just as we do.

Most humans find it incredibly difficult (if not impossible) to sit quietly and simply be 'in the moment' with you. They have a permanent need for noise, or visual diversion. (By this I mean phone scrolling, booming background music, a blaring television, burbling radio, or being with other humans.) They also suffer from touch diversion which involves patting or stroking you very quickly, smoking, vaping, eating, drinking, or just general hand-fidgeting.

None of this behaviour is calming or connecting. In truth, it's the complete opposite. It's creating a diversion and NOT connecting with you.

Their frenetic lives have a knock-on effect to you, especially if you're a particularly gentle soul, or from a breed known for its super-intelligence and sensitivity. I'm thinking Poodles and Collies.

Humans find it hard to be still and serene

By calm connection, I mean that you and your human share a quiet 10 or 15 minutes, undisturbed. In reality, this means your human isn't doing anything, not one thing. They are simply 'being' with you, calmly and quietly. It's not something many humans do, and the idea of sitting with you and doing nothing will be a most alien concept to many of them. If you're able to influence or encourage them in any way, I highly recommend you do so, for both your benefits.

Humans know you live in the moment, but as I've said previously, largely, they do not. Taking just a short time out of their day to be 'in the moment' with you will be a very loving experience for you both. Ideally, they should simply sit with you, whether it's on the floor beside your bed, on the sofa – if you're allowed – on the lawn, the patio, or even stopping on a bench or by a river when out for a walk.

Touching you very slowly and quietly is an excellent way for them to connect with you and to strengthen your mutual bond. You will love to share their serenity if they put a halt to their ever-whirling minds and tune into their true selves. It's highly likely they will enjoy it too.

The big challenge here for your human is doing nothing for 10 minutes. Humans call this mindfulness. I call it calm connection with their canine (that's you.) It's by and large being mindful with you and in my opinion, there's nowhere near enough of it in this chaotic human (and canine) world.

Professor Daniel's Bones of Retention:

- **You sense things humans don't**
- **Sad humans need your waggy tail**
- **Avoid angry or aggressive people**
- **Human-hound goals forge strong bonds**
- **Stressed humans create stressed dogs**
- **Sharing joy with your human is special**
- **Calm connection is the best medicine**

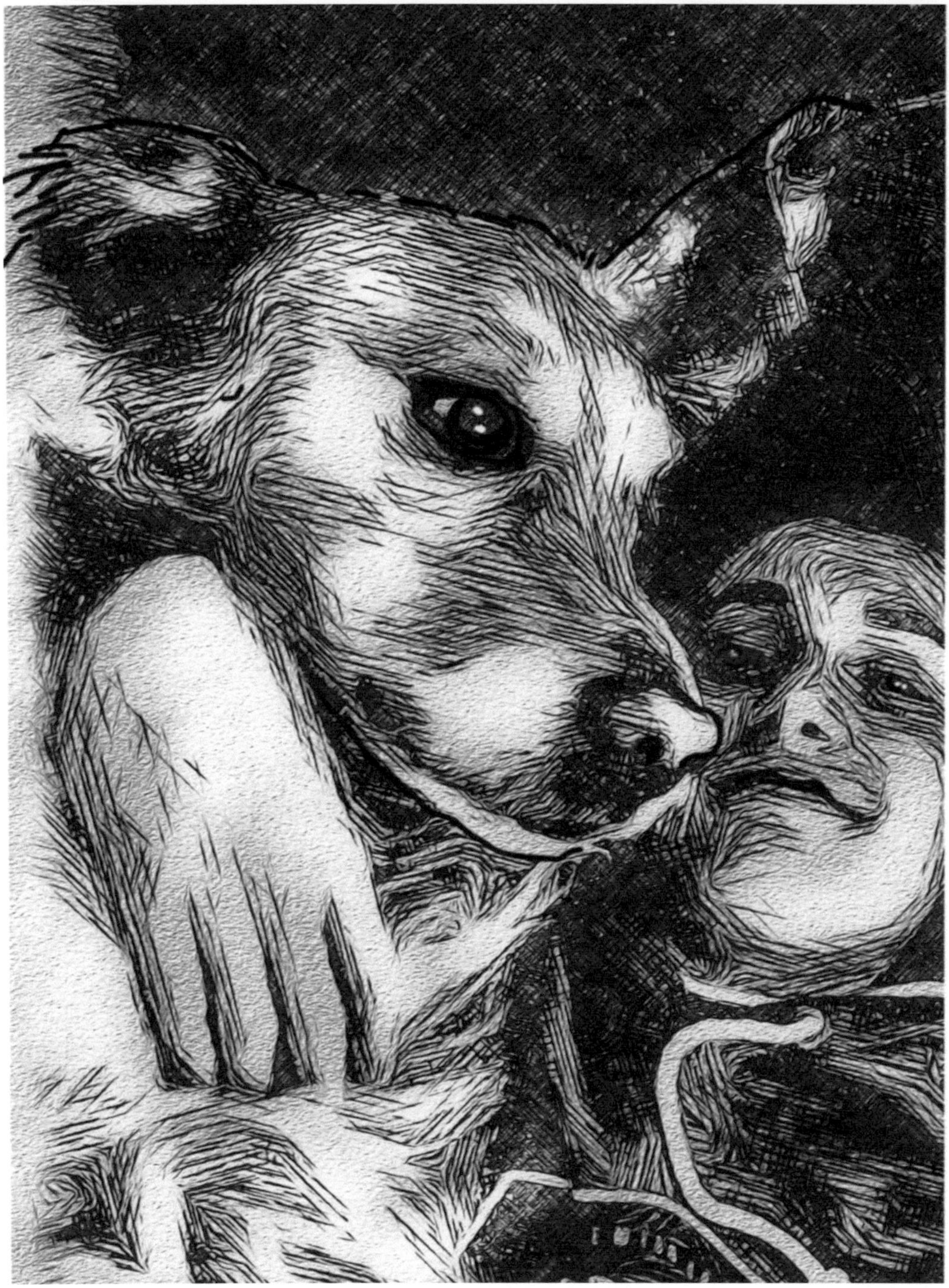

"We need more calm connection between humans and their canines in this chaotic world."

Chapter 4

Humans with high-speed lives

When joining a human home, you'll find their lives are often frantic and busy. These humans haven't yet learned to curb their urge to whirl and worry, reel and rush, strive and stress.

Their lives are lived at high-speed, giving out a rough and tumble vibe, full of noise and natter. It's a high-arousal environment and if there's no down time, it can spell doggy disaster for your mental and physical health.

Unfortunately, so busy are these high-speed humans leading their high-speed lives, they may not have the time to consider its effect on you. The simple truth is this sort of lifestyle does you absolutely no doggy good whatsoever.

You'll join in of course and it's likely no one will be any the wiser. You'll be up, down, in and out, revved up and racing around (just like them), while being bombarded by all manner of household noise and human kerfuffle.

It's likely you'll join in this holy hullabaloo by proudly carrying around shoes and slippers at the drop of a, well, shoe. You'll have your head in any school bags, handbags or shopping bags that touch the floor and you'll be cavorting up and down stairs, in and out of the garden like a doggie version of Mo Farrah – but with four legs obviously and a little slower.

However, due to your extremely sensitive nature, you must guard against absorbing too much of their hot-headed hoo-ha. If you live in a frantic household with one or more high-speed humans, you must be on your guard. By frantic household, I mean one that behaves as if they're in a noisy, aggression-fuelled television soap opera. They may thrive on and create at least one crisis a day, more if you're unlucky. The chances are your humans will have not the slightest canine clue the effect their 'drama-llama' lives have on you.

I have met dozens of dogs who have become jabbering, anxious wrecks from soaking up the mental turmoil of their high-speed humans. If you live in such a home, I suggest you keep your head on your paws, your eyes shut, ears down and spend as much time outdoors as you can.

High-speed humans create high-speed dogs

Some of these high-speed humans are likely to buy you a ball which they throw repeatedly, or toys to tug them off their feet. These activities are fun and of course you throw yourself into them with doggy gusto, enjoying the attention. (It may be the only direct human-time you receive in their hectic household, so understandably you take what you can.) As born people-pleasers you want to make your human happy. You will revel in their praise when you return said ball, or tug said tugger.

But, if this high-energy interaction is all you receive from your human, it's extremely unhealthy for you and the chances are, you will become a dog that is unable to switch off or relax. Just like your humans, you will be worrying, whirling and looking for the next distraction or diversion.

As I say, living in this high-speed home of man-made commotion will take its toll on a sensitive soul like you. One day you'll wake up feeling not quite so bouncy and full of the joys, you may even feel a little anxious, without really knowing why. This emotional tension can creep up on a canine like a stealthy cat and before you know it, you are in the grip of its needle-like claws with anxiety as your new, unwanted friend.

By the time your humans notice you're not your usual joyful, balanced doggy self, the emotional damage is already setting in. Your previous happy-go-lucky approach to life is becoming one of fearful trepidation. Your anxiety levels are rising, you begin barking at random visitors and other dogs.

Rather than spending the evening on the sofa with your humans, you take yourself off to a quiet corner, preferring to be alone in another part of the house. You may refuse to go out for a walk, preferring the security of your garden. If you do go out, you'll probably want to stay close to your human (safety in numbers); you may want to remain on the lead, rather than risk the scary scenario of meeting other dogs. Your world becomes a worrying place - not unlike the frenzied one in which your humans live.

Balls and sticks can make you sick

As I've mentioned, one of the diversions your hurried human may offer you, is the ball thrower game. This is where they take you to a field or park every day for your exercise, with a plastic scoop in which sits a ball. This long-handled hurler is repeatedly launched sky-ward, sending the ball hurtling across the park or field. What will you do? You will, of course, race as fast as your little legs will carry you to retrieve it. Possibly leaping, twisting and jumping at great speed in the process.

I know many of you love playing ball. But, as far as these throwers are concerned, I'm afraid it's bad news. This high impact, repetitive play really isn't good for you. (The only good repetitive actions are eating, digging and mating – and they don't last long.)

Take it from me - you aren't a ballerina, gymnast, contortionist or even an Olympic high-jumper. Your bodies simply aren't built to run continuously at speed, back and forth, twisting and jumping after a ball, hour after hour, day after day. I've heard of many a vet dealing with broken toes, torn cruciate ligaments and sprained shoulders, thanks to humans wielding these wicked throwers as far as their biceps allow. I've seen dogs tear off after their balls like demented whirling dervishes, oblivious to every man and beast in their path, eyes firmly focused only on that brightly-coloured bouncy-ball target.

These humans are very well-meaning but probably oblivious to the risks. They think it's good exercise to tire you out like this every day. It's not. The only thing it's good for, is damaging and weakening your joints, inviting in early arthritis and injury. There are also biological and emotional prices you pay for this unnatural exercise. I implore you (and any of your humans who may read this) to give it a miss.

Canines weren't created for this type of high-performance, athletic activity. It's not a sport in which you should indulge on a prolonged, daily basis. It should be viewed as an occasional treat, maybe once or twice a week for a few minutes at a time.

Like any habit, if carried out daily, week in, week out, it becomes like a drug to you, similar to humans with their various addictions. You run the risk of becoming ball-obsessed, thinking only of that bouncy round reward. If you don't get your ball fix, you're likely to become demanding, stressed, aggressive even, or reactive. Humans probably won't understand what's going on when you bark or whine for more. Keen to appease you, they will give in to your demands, thinking it's pure fun and enjoyment that drives you on. They don't realise it's actually a ball-crazed, adrenalin-fuelled, manic state. It's not so dissimilar to a human drug addict shouting for more of their substance.

Every time you play ball your body is flooded with adrenalin and it stays in your system for hours afterwards. If ball-chasing is your everyday exercise, your system is never free from those fight or flight hormones – so your delicate doggy mind never gets the opportunity to switch off.

Case study: Libby the Labradoodle

Libby is 6-years-old and is recovering from a snapped cruciate ligament. She's also been diagnosed with early-onset arthritis in her front legs. Her human, Roger, took Libby to the park every day with a ball thrower. Libby admitted to Dr Peter Pointer that her desire to please her dad ended in serious injury for her and worry and expense for her dad.

"I love the park, I love balls, and of course I love my dad. Put the three together and it was heaven. That was until I noticed my legs feeling a bit sore at the end of the day. I'm half Labrador Retriever, so of course if Dad threw a ball, I'd go and fetch it for him. And my goodness! He threw it such a long way with that plastic stick. Even

when my tongue was hanging out, my eyes couldn't focus and my legs were almost buckling beneath me, Dad kept on throwing that ball so of course, I kept retrieving it for him. I'd have done it until I collapsed because all I wanted to do was please my dad. Sometimes he'd even do it in the summer, when I'd really rather lie on the cool grass under a tree. But he's my dad and I love him, so of course I did it for him.

"One day we'd been playing ball for half an hour. I'd been jumping, skidding, chasing and turning. It was our second session of the day. As I twisted to try to catch the ball, I felt something snap in my back leg. It was agony and I couldn't put any weight on it. Dad was very worried and carried me straight to the vets. I'm now recovering from what Dad said was very expensive surgery. I am on restricted lead walks for 12 - 16 weeks. My leg is very sore and painful. The x-rays also showed my joints were inflamed. I tried to tell Dad that some time ago. I'd lie down in the park when my legs were sore, but he kept throwing the ball for me to fetch and urging me on. This is what can happen when you fetch the ball for your human every day. I wish the thrower had snapped instead of my leg. I'm hoping when I'm better, we can just have some walks around the park or in the woods that I can enjoy at my own pace."

Beware sticks that behave like spears

Now, as well as protecting your delicate doggy joints, there's another similar habit you really shouldn't develop - and that's chasing and retrieving sticks. I know, I know, dogs and sticks are like salt and pepper, they tend to go together, especially if you're a working breed. In the past, I've seen highly-wired Collies, very proud Labradors, and delighted Spaniels (and various hybrids) pouncing on, retrieving and even carrying aloft impressively large sticks of tree-like proportions.

Now the carrying of the bark-shredded stick isn't the problem. There's nothing better for some of you than carrying an exceptionally wide load of a stick in true, tight-rope walker style. Part of the fun is of course crashing into everything and everyone in your path (human legs and ankles included).

The danger lurks when your human hurls a stick of the shorter, pointier variety across a field, or park. You hare after it like some demented tree devil on four legs and as it lands, spear-like into the ground, you're in danger of charging headlong onto it, jamming it down your throat. Reminiscent of a hounds of hell horror film, you will be screaming in pain, blood pouring from your fangs as the stick points arrow-like from your oesophagus. Your human is of course in full panic mode, knowing not whether to leave the stick in, or pull it out, but is fully aware this is an emergency, rush-to-the-vet NOW situation.

Case study: Weaver the Golden Retriever

Dr Peter Pointer knew Weaver personally. He was involved in a sickening 'sticky' situation and it was an horrendous ordeal for both Weaver and his human. Here's his story:

"I was out walking with my young mum, a teenager, who looked after me very well," recalled Weaver. "Being a Retriever, I loved to fetch things. Mum knew this and usually found a stick to throw for me. On this fateful day, the stick Mum found had a rather pointed end and a tendency to split. She threw it quite a way and I sped after it in my usual eager fashion. Unfortunately for me, the stick

landed like a javelin. As I grabbed the end, I misjudged the distance and it slid down the back of my throat. The pain was awful and I screamed. I could feel this piece of wood stuck fast down my throat and could taste blood in my mouth. I collapsed on the floor and Mum came running up, shouting my name. She carefully pulled the stick out, but I couldn't stand up. I'm not sure to this day if it was the shock, the pain, or what. Poor Mum was crying and although only a slight thing, she heaved me up into her arms and carried me, staggering back home. There were no mobile phones in those days. I was taken to the vet, who discovered the stick had splintered and pieces of it were embedded deep down into my throat in various places. I underwent surgery to remove them. We didn't know it at the time, but not all the splinters were removed that day. Those that remained became infected. I had many more trips to the vet and surgery and sported an open wound on my chest which constantly oozed smelly pus. Eventually, I was referred to Bristol vet college where a team of student vets used me as a 'sticky' case study. Thankfully for me, they were able to remove the rest of the splinters and the chest wound healed, as did my throat. But it took a long time - and Mum never threw a stick for me again."

You're not natural runners

Now you'll find many humans enjoy repetition, especially when it comes to exercise. One repetitive sport that your human may want you to undertake, is running. (This is usually because that's what they like to do.)

Even in our dim and distance past, our ancestors didn't run non-stop for five, ten, or 15 miles. Short, high-speed chases of prey, or fleeing for our lives from a predator were more our thing.

Some breeds are natural racers. Greyhounds and whippets of course, but they run very quickly in incredibly short bursts. Trailhounds race at their own speed over 10-mile aniseed trails, while Foxhounds career around the countryside with horses following scents. If you're a working Spaniel, Labrador, or Collie, slightly different rules apply. But even then, you're unlikely to be running continuously; there will be breaks of sitting and waiting.

It's rare to find a non-working dog that takes itself off to run non-stop simply for the sake and enjoyment of it – but it's something humans do. They do it for fitness and competitive events. The issue is, they may want to take you along too. Much like with ball-throwers, most of you aren't built for non-stop, long-distance running. Your ideal exercise is running or playing chase with other canine friends for the fun of it and in shorter bursts.

For most of you, your walk should be predominantly that, a walk. It's a chance for you to sniff, snuffle, investigate, delve and dig. To run at your own pace, on your own terms, not at a frenetic pace driven by a ball, or a human in running kit.

A walk is an opportunity for your human to connect with you and their surroundings. Sadly, many humans do not appreciate, or do this. Rather than watching your antics, taking an interest in your investigations, they will more likely be engrossed with human diversions. They will be on their phones (again), listening to music through ear pods, or engrossed in chat with another human. Walking while being diverted is not being in the moment, in nature or connecting. It's another example of humans not being in and enjoying the here and now as you do.

Grounded humans are good for you

Humans don't realise we are adversely affected by all this extraneous entertainment. Really, all we need for the good of our doggy health, is some peace and quiet. Most of them probably do too, if truth be told. My experience shows that if you are lucky enough to live with humans who value nature and the outdoor life, you will enjoy a calmer, more grounded existence too.

As nature intended, is a human phrase, but it goes for you too. Like all animals, we canines were born in the wild and although domesticated thousands of years ago, we still carry some of those instincts. Don't misunderstand me - we love sharing our lives with humans. Out of all the species, we are the ones who chose to be close to them. Our problem is that homo sapiens are now so far removed from their own natural roots, it has widened the gap between us – to both of our detriments.

Case study: Womble the Working Cocker

Womble the Working Cocker goes running with his human Mandy. She wears earplugs with music coursing through them. Womble runs dutifully alongside Mandy. He told Dr Peter Pointer these were the only 'walks' he had.

"I love running and I love being with my mum. But what I would love more, is to snuffle in the hedgerows and ditches, put up pheasants and chase around in circles on deer scents. I'm only

allowed to pause on our run for a pee or a poo, then Mum whistles me to hurry up and get running again. Sometimes my paws feel a bit sore, as we run on the road quite a bit. My legs also get tired. There are so many sniffs I'd like to explore, but I'm not allowed. I have to keep up with Mum. Once, I couldn't help disappearing into a ditch where I knew a pheasant was hiding. I was barking frantically to tell Mum what I'd found - I was very excited. She couldn't hear me with her earplugs in and it was quite some time before she realised I hadn't caught up. She wasn't best pleased with me, but I was very happy snuffling about in my ditch. I was bred to snuffle, not to jog."

Re-connecting with us and nature is a very hard lesson to teach your human. I know many of you have suffered deeply in the trying. Taking on some of their stress and anxiety and shouldering some of the burdens they carry, is very noble. It demonstrates your unconditional love for your human. But it comes at a canine cost, because absorbing the stress of their frantic lives can make you ill.

Professor Daniel's Bones of Retention:

- **Human lives can be frantic**
- **Ball throwers are your worst friends**
- **Encourage your human to 'just be'**
- **Chasing sticks is a risky pastime**
- **Adrenalin play is addictive**
- **You're not a long-distance runner***
- **If you're over-exercised, lie down**

***Working dog exclusions apply**

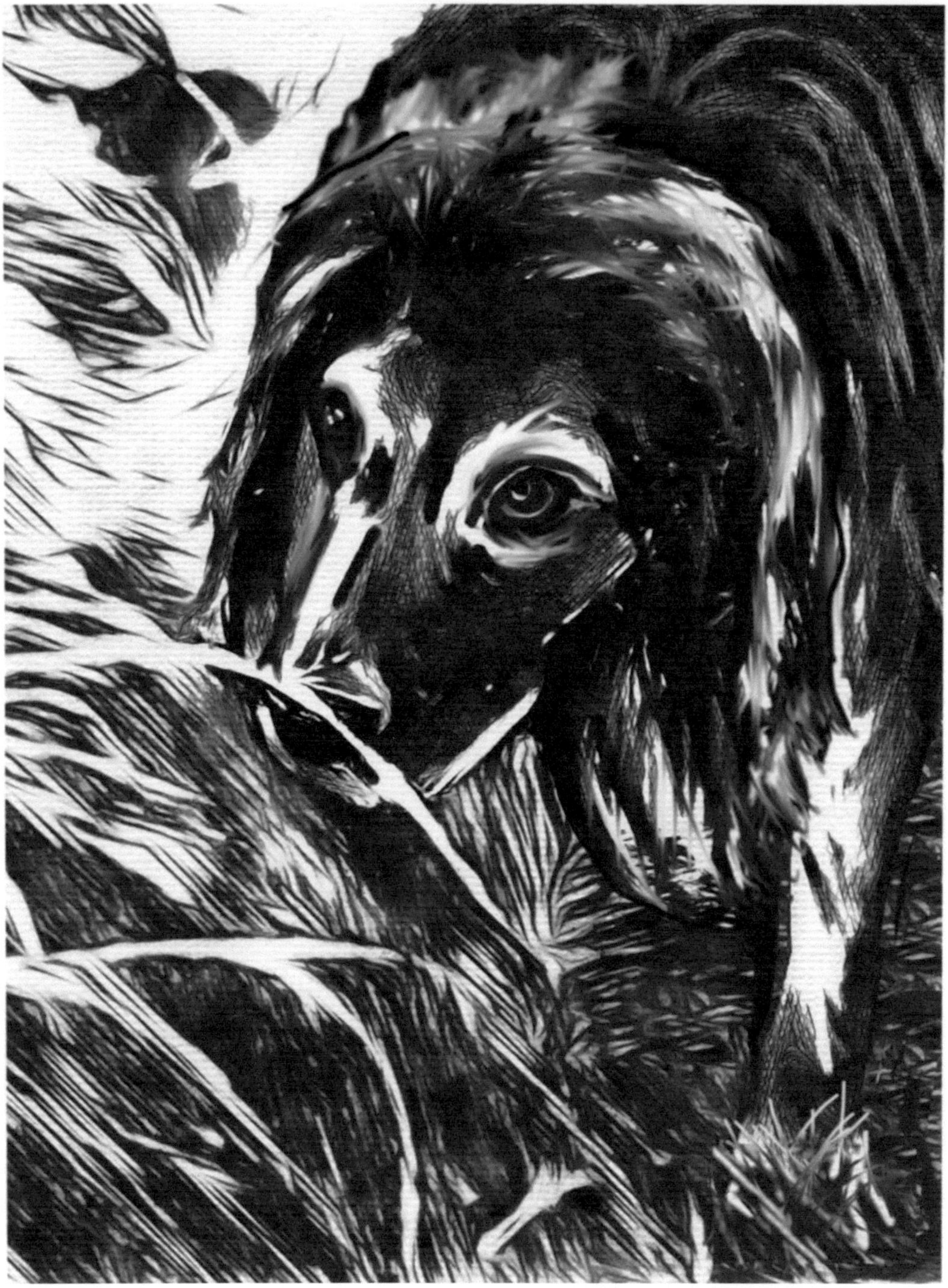

"A walk should be a chance to sniff, snuffle and investigate at your own pace."

Chapter 5

Types of humans: Love seekers

During your lifetime, you're going to come across all sorts of weird and wonderful humans. Now I'm hoping that the human you begin your life with (and paws crossed it's a long and happy one at that) is the same one who supports you at the end.

Unfortunately, for a multitude of reasons, due to the foibles of the human world, this isn't always the case. But of one thing I can be sure. You will meet some humans who recoil in disdain from your loving licks and nose nudges. Don't take it personally, there's obviously something very wrong with them.

There will be others who go out of their way to say hello to you because you are so beautifully appealing. Some will roll around on the floor cuddling and playing with you, caring not a bit as their mouth fills with your hair and their clothes are covered in your fur. (The last two human types are the ones to choose if you can.)

As far as I can see humans fall into four broad categories. I stress broad because some humans may be hybrids and of course, there are exceptions to every rule.

The first type of human is the love seeker - that's one who simply wants something furry to love. These humans are indeed very sweet and loving, but may lack a few brain cells. (That's even less than the average human.) The love seeker will put your needs above all else. This is to be admired, but do heed this woof of warning. In extreme cases, they will treat you like a human and there's a risk of you being killed by kindness.

This may seem fun at first, especially at Christmas when you're served up roast turkey, gravy and all the fatty trimmings. But when you're dashing to the back door with colitis at 1 am, complete with a trail of foul-smelling diarrhoea behind you, it's no fun at all. Your human won't think so either.

Similarly, in a drunken late-night haze, your human may think "itzz a grreat ideya" to feed their little 'fur-baby' some of their rich and yummy cheesy dip. It will definitely go down very well with you at the time, but mark my words, it will come back up just as easily at 6 am the next day, on their favourite fluffy mat. Some hours later, when your human finally surfaces, hungover, head-in-hands, they'll no doubt pad barefoot straight into your strategically-placed, pile of vomit. Seeing, feeling and smelling regurgitated cheesy dip between their toes won't win you any brownie points - or cheesy ones either for that matter.

Of course, inappropriate gorging on human goodies is not actually your fault. If your human feeds you dogilicious delicacies that are actually unfit for your doggy digestion, that's their lookout. It's rare to find a dog who holds up a paw to refuse a tasty titbit, fearing it will give them indigestion or make them sick. Having a gurgly tummy, smelly flatulence and occasional vomiting are part and parcel of being a dog. Eat first, eject later, is your motto in that respect. In many cases, the ejection comes because you've scoffed something too quickly, or have eaten food that you shouldn't have touched in the first place. But if a human treats your belly with the same gung-ho attitude as they do their own, it does you no foodie favours at all.

Blurring your boundaries is bad news

There are other doggy drawbacks to being treated as a human. Blurring the line between their behaviour and yours is unhealthy and I'd go as far as to say, unsafe. You end up living in a baffling betwixt world as a sort of HuDog. This means that although a canine at heart, you're encouraged by your human to act and live like homo-sapiens. This homo-hound life is both confusing and potentially damaging to your delicate doggy demeanour. You have the natural instincts of a dog, but you're living as a human. You could find yourself wearing all sorts of unnecessary designer coats and seasonal outfits. You may have your own place setting at meal times or be carried around in a bag or pushchair. It's unlikely any self-respecting canine harbours a desire to dress up, eat at a table or be airborne. Having all four paws on terra firma is your natural state. But alas, your love-seeking human may have other ideas, more often to please themselves than you. In time, if you're subjected to this sort of humanising on a regular basis you may start to believe you are one (may Dog-God preserve us).

You can end up as co-dependent on your human and vice-versa and that's not a happy place for a hound to be. A HuDog life can lead to you displaying neurotic and even reactive behaviour. You may feel overwhelmed, unsure, baffled and anxious. You need constant reassurance from your human because the world is overwhelming. You can no longer relate to your doggy friends and become fearful and anti-social in the canine world. These feelings are from living as a HuDog and again, it's through no fault of your own.

Love seekers enjoy your attention

Now love seekers are the humans most at risk of turning you into a HuDog. This is because they are most likely to set you no healthy boundaries. (You'll read about boundaries in Chapter 9.) You could well be a HuDog if you ask your human for fuss by continually jumping up or pawing at them, whining or barking at them. Despite this rather immature behaviour, 99 per cent of the time you'll get what you want, regardless of what your human is doing. In fact, if you're a HuDog you'll be allowed to jump up at your human whenever and wherever you please. It matters not if they're sitting down reading, snoozing, watching television, enjoying a glass of wine or chatting with friends. As long as you make a big enough nuisance of yourself, you'll get that pat, stroke or belly rub.

Some humans see this behaviour as a sign of how much you love them. There is no doubt whatsoever that you love them. You love them to bits, unconditionally. That's what we dogs do. So, while there is some truth in this, I believe the over-riding reason for your behaviour is that as a HuDog, your 'Dog Off' button no longer works, because your love seeker has inadvertently switched it off.

The Dog Off button is your natural instinct that tells you all is well with the world. It says you're safe and secure and it's quite ok to take yourself off to a quiet corner for a lie down and a sleep. In the wild days of old, it would have been your rest and digest time, after a good feed. The time when you relax, unwind and watch the world go with a full belly and sleepy eyes. For our wolf cousins, if food was plentiful, that was a substantial amount of the time.

However, today's HuDogs usually spend a lot of their day on the go; even when resting they are on the alert, ready to spring into action or bark at the slightest opportunity, for they cannot switch off.

Case study: Lindy-Lou the Cockapoo

Lindy-Lou is unable to sit quietly on her own or feel relaxed around other dogs. She told Dr Peter Pointer she only feels safe when sitting on her Mum's lap, lying at her feet or when she's touching her.

She says: *"I love sitting on Mum and having her fuss me. I'm pretty sure she loves it too. She's let me climb on her since I was a pup and always gives me her full attention, whether she's alone, with family or friends. Sometimes she gently pushes me away and tells me to get down, but I know she doesn't mean it. Her voice is very soft and not at all stern. I know if I carry on making a bit of a nuisance of myself, she'll give in and I'll get what I want. I always do. I'm happy when I'm touching Mum because I feel safe then. I'm uneasy if she's not touching me. Most dogs love a walk but they make me feel anxious. I'm not comfortable outside and I don't like seeing other dogs, so hide behind Mum and shake. I only feel relaxed when Mum's petting me."*

HuDogs often feel anxious

Lindy-Lou's case is a prime example of how treating you like a HuDog, can encourage you to behave anti-socially. You become a dog who doesn't fit easily into the canine world. The

HuDog's existence can quickly become a dog's dinner of a life, with serious behavioural issues. That's you with the issues not the human, although it could be argued one is intertwined with the other!

You may find love seekers rely on you for their own emotional support and turn to you in times of trouble. You may find your fur absolutely soaked by tears as your human hangs on to you for dear life, after a difficult experience. They will tell you in detail about their dashed career hopes, their life fears and loves lost. That's OK for a short time, and after all, if a human can't confide in us canines, who can they talk to? But, if this becomes a daily habit and begins to consume their (and your) lives, you'll need to take things into your own paws.

Once you've extricated yourself from their vice-like grip, try standing by the door and whining. If you're of the Retriever variety, fetch your lead. A good walk will help clear their heads and give you a bit of breathing space. If they want to spend all day in their pyjamas, eating chocolate with the telly on, bark loudly and ask to go in the garden. Watch the birds and catch the flies, sniff out any visiting wildlife, have a wee and dig a big hole to relieve your frustration. There's nothing like a good dig to calm a disturbed doggie mind. It should also divert their attention back to you and your needs, rather than focusing purely on their own. Some humans can be quite selfish like that.

If that behaviour fails, pull apart one of your toys, or play with a squeaky one. Make a general nuisance of yourself. If desperate measures are needed (and I wouldn't condone this), you may consider chewing up something of theirs – a slipper, a hat, the telly remote or their prized possession, their mobile phone. I would never encourage such anti-social behaviour, but I understand how, when driven to distraction by your human's actions, or lack of them, it may be your last resort as all other options have failed.

A less destructive solution, is to perhaps just run about with said possession in your mouth - rather than destroying it. Or just sit and look longingly out of the window, or scratch at the door. With a bit more Lassie luck, your self-pitying human will get the message, put some clothes on and take you for a walk. It will do them the world of good too.

Case study: Diesel the Dachshund

As a pup Diesel was tiny. Even when fully-grown, he was very low to the ground. He told Dr Peter Pointer that he was rarely allowed to walk by himself. He was his human's first dog.

Diesel says: *"I think Mum viewed me as a precious doll rather than a dog. She would dress me up in outfits. I had a yellow mac for when it rained, a cooling vest for warmer weather and a whole wardrobe of other tops and coats. To be honest, I felt quite uncomfortable in them. I was quite content with my fur, but it was what Mum wanted, so of course I went along with it, letting her put my paws into the sleeve holes. As a pup, she insisted on carrying me most of the time. I was only allowed to walk on the ground if there were no other dogs around. If she saw one in the distance, she would hurriedly pick me up. She was scared the other dogs would hurt me because I'm small. In truth, I wasn't scared of my fellow canines. I was curious and wanted to sniff, meet and socialise with them. I wasn't worried about their size. But every time I saw another potential playmate, Mum scooped me up in her arms. She was scared and I felt her fear. This happened on all our walks, so I wasn't allowed to meet, greet or make any furry friends. As the months went by, and following Mum's lead, I became scared of other dogs too. As I grew, my fear grew. To support Mum, I would bark at any dogs who came near us, to warn them off. On the odd occasion we were taken by surprise and I'd meet a dog while I was on the ground. Immediately, I sensed Mum's fear so I would snarl and bark at them, keeping them away just as Mum had taught me. She didn't want them near us and, by then, neither did I."*

A HuDog is generally an unhappy dog that's uncomfortable in its own furry skin. Being a HuDog robs you of displaying your natural canine behaviour and of feeling at ease in your environment. It's not a healthy place for you to be and to change it, professional help and guidance may be needed.

Professor Daniel's Bones of Retention

- **Love seekers can kill you with kindness**
- **You are NOT a human**
- **Homo-hound life is unhealthy**
- **Some humans are selfish**
- **A walk clears a human head (and yours)**
- **Dig a hole if you feel frustrated**
- **HuDogs are unhappy dogs**

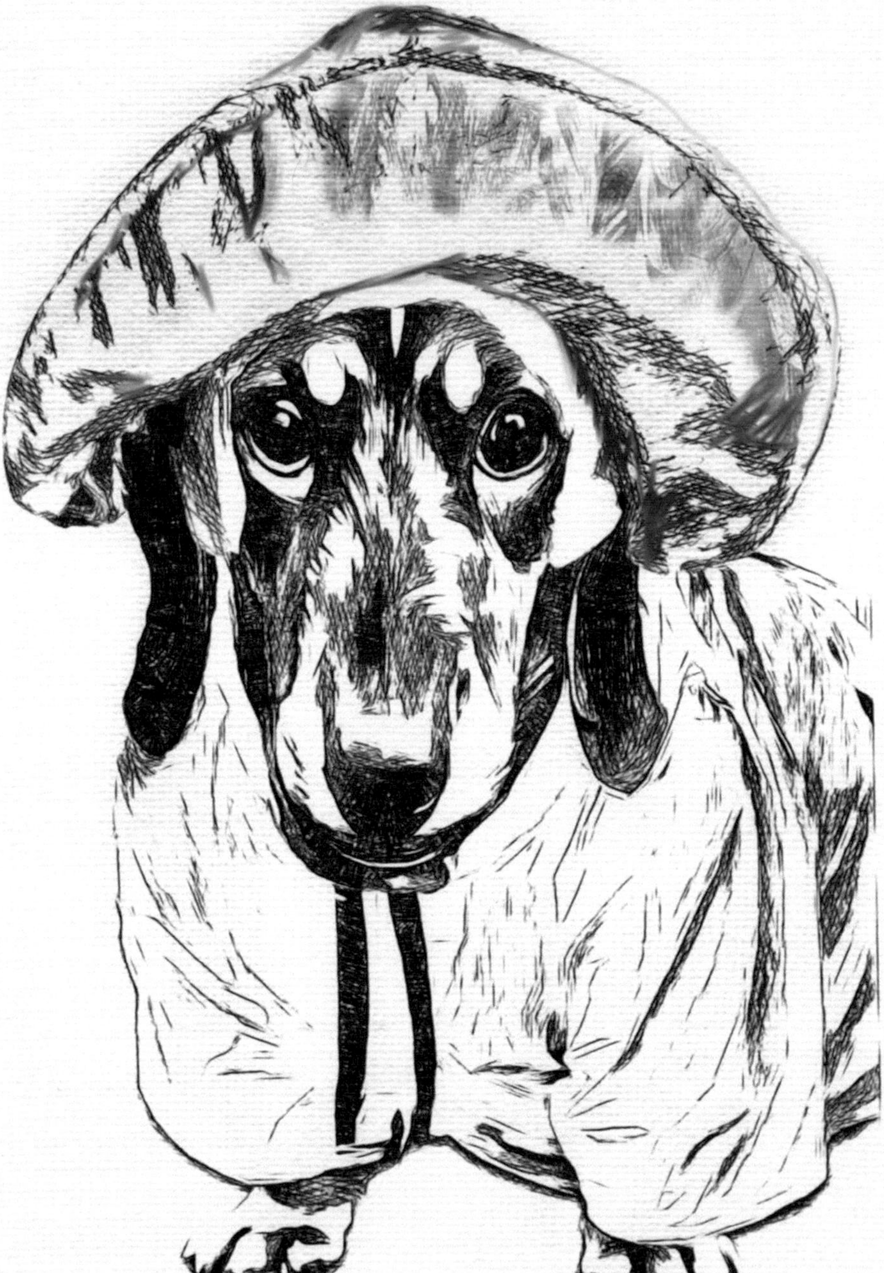

"A canine at heart, you are encouraged to live like a human in a baffling betwixt world."

Chapter 6

Types of humans: Impulse buyers

These humans think owning a dog will be fun and lovely. While you are certainly a fun and lovely addition to any life, these humans don't stop to consider what your many needs are, or how they will meet them.

Unfortunately, you're unlikely to have any say in this, so there's very little you can do to change it. These humans fall into two categories: The first are the selfish impulse buyers. These are the more self-centred humans who want you simply to satisfy their whims. Their decision to get you is likely to be more akin to buying a new pair of shoes, or a sofa. The only thought that goes into it is the enjoyment and pleasure they hope to gain from you. I believe very little, if any thought, is given to your future needs. They may buy you as a pup from a breeder who doesn't ask too many questions and demands a high price for the privilege.

The second category of impulse buyers are those who lack common sense. Though kind and loving, they haven't researched or thought through the practical or logistical implications of having you in their life and ultimately, you're the one who suffers.

In my view the rather selfish impulse buyer would be better off buying themselves a stuffed toy. Through their rose-tinted, doggy-shaped glasses, they see you skipping happily at their side through sunshine-filled fields sniffing flowers and waving a friendly paw to the grazing sheep and lambs. They are expecting a bit of a furry fairy tale but are more likely to end up in a nail-biting nightmare.

Their fanciful expectations of dog ownership are completely at odds with the reality of having you share their homes and lives. They are surprised to discover that you're not content to sit quietly all day on your own while they're at work. They're also shocked to learn that, unlike a pretty ornament, you need a lot of time, patience, commitment, dedication, training and exercise. These humans really are barking up the wrong tree – and there's no one better placed than us to advise on trees and barking.

The simple fact is that these types of humans who decide to share their lives with you, need educating. The impulse buyers view you as more of a play thing or accessory. They think you will slot into their lives quite easily - and these are lives which are, more often than not, already busy and sometimes hectic. Once living in their home, they will find you can't be stuffed back into the box – even if you are a Terrier called Jack.

Impulse buyers don't consider your needs

My studies have unearthed countless canines who have ended up in the most unsuitable hands after humans have bought them either on a whim, or without applying one iota of common sense.

I've been told sad tales of Labradors or Pointers living in cramped, first-floor flats with no outdoor space. I've seen Collies driven to distraction after being confined to a two-roomed home. I've met Miniature Dachshunds whose days were spent sitting in handbags like a piece of living jewellery.

I've seen others of you confined to wire crates for eight hours a day, while your humans are at work. You could be forgiven for feeling like a dejected exhibit in a zoo, or an inmate in a high-security dog jail. You really should not be subjected to such treatment. My guess is it's because you're viewed as being 'just a dog' rather than a sentient being. Even humans living in a prison are given daily exercise and stimulation during their day. I can't imagine your human would enjoy sitting in a cage for hour after hour, without company, or a chance to stretch their legs.

When your human does return home at the end of their long working day, understandably, you will be extremely pleased to see them. You may wee on the floor, or on them, running around wildly out-of-control. Some of you will be so delighted to have their company, you will be jumping up and down at your humans in energetic, trampoline-fashion, scratching them or their special work clothes in the process. (Many a human's pair of tights has been laddered and smart suit hair-smothered, by a lonely canine welcoming home its human family.) Young children may be sent flying and crying and prized rugs, jugs and other objets d'arts may suffer a similar fate.

Your humans may term your behaviour mad, or bad. Some will say it is because you are pleased to see them (which you are of course), but they're likely to overlook the fact that the main driver for your supposedly barmy behaviour is down to lack of company, stimulation and exercise.

You may never run free off-lead

These humans are probably the very same ones who term a walk as a quick stroll around the local park. In this instance, you'll find yourself on a tight, short lead, or at the end of the long, retractable one. It's possible you won't ever be allowed to run loose and enjoy your freedom because these humans fear losing you - because they've not trained you. I accept it's a strong possibility that you may run off - or not do as you're asked. This is only because they won't have shown you the behaviour they'd like from you – known to humans as dog training.

If your impulse buyer works full-time, they will soon discover they can't find time to walk you, let alone train you. Had they done their research, they'd have learnt that training and socialising you as a pup, is vital to you growing up to be a happy and balanced girl, boy, or anything else you may be in between.

As a result of their lack of knowledge, your life is restricted to being outdoors on a lead for perhaps 15 minutes a day, a few metres from their feet. Full of frustration, you'll be pulling like a train, eager to burn off your pent-up energy. If you're confined to barracks all day, you'll probably be feeling lonely and neglected too. When you do finally get your 15-minutes of furry, outdoor fame, you'll be desperate to meet other canines. Alas, I'm afraid your ill-educated impulse buyer will have other ideas.

Unable to contain your exuberance (the result of no time to train or socialise), your human is likely to do one of two things.

Firstly, they may steer clear of you passing the time of day with other canines by completely avoiding their presence. This means you don't get the opportunity to socialise with other dogs and you risk growing up to be either, anxious and recoiling, or fearful and aggressive.

The second possibility is that you will be allowed to pull them along in your wake as you charge up to any dog you see - whether the other dog wants to see you or not. This action has other repercussions. If the other dog is off-lead, you may get away with your uninvited approaches, because it's free to move away from you. If it's happy to meet you, your human will probably be jerked off their feet as you try to chase and play. A jolted shoulder or strained back later, your human will be calling the chiropractor once they return home.

If you are on a long, retractable lead (I call these LAPATTs the LAzy Person's Alternative To Training), I can guarantee you'll end up in one gigantic jumble. The thin, nylon cord also runs a high risk of cutting tightly and painfully into any available human legs. There will be much circling of people, raising of arms and unravelling of cord, in a doggy dance not dissimilar to 'round and round the mulberry bush'. This human-hound hubbub will be accompanied by a rhythmical clicking of plastic. This provides the background beat as your human desperately tries to avoid bright red nylon cord burns as you attempt to play with your new friend while still tethered.

Greeting other dogs uninvited is risky

However, a different story may unfold, if your new friend is still on his or her lead. If your human allows you to go bounding up to a dog uninvited, the situation could go one of several ways. If the other dog is anxious or reactive, you're quite possibly bounding headlong into a fight. Your unrestrained eagerness to say hello (and your human's lack of common sense), means you are likely to be greeted with a warning snarl, a vicious snapping of teeth, or a clamping-on of jaws. You'll be caught completely off-guard, returning home with at least a puncture wound or two. Worst case scenario is a vet visit for stitches to a nasty bite and injections to quell the pain and stop infection.

Your rather naive human hadn't considered that the other dog may be unsocialised, fearful of other canines or even recovering from surgery. Elderly dogs and those with arthritis, a weak spine or other health conditions often feel vulnerable among energetic young dogs. Their only way to protect themselves from further pain (from you) is to react or attack. If your human allows you to go charging in, the poor dog could end up in a sorrier state. You jumping eagerly on its back asking to play won't be well-received. Your human could find themselves not only berated by the other dog's angry owner, but also presented with a hefty vet bill for the bodily damage you may have inadvertently inflicted by your boisterous bouncings.

Case study: Ollie the Sprollie (Collie cross Springer)

Ollie the Sprollie was bought by his dad, a man in his 70s, as a companion after he lost his wife of 50 years. His dad hadn't owned a working breed before, he hadn't researched it at all and was completely out of his depth. Ollie talked through his frustrations with Dr Peter Pointer.

Ollie says: "My dad is a very kind man and I love him very much. But I really want to run my legs off in the field, chasing pheasants and sniffing the hedgerows. That's what my doggy mum and dad both did. My dad only has a small garden and it's got strange plastic grass that doesn't smell or feel right. He's not done any training with me, so I don't know how he wants me to behave. He says I'm a bright boy and I'd love to learn but he doesn't teach me anything.

"We go on walks, but he keeps me on a long lead. I've got a lot of energy, so in my excitement at being outside, I jump about and pull him around a lot. Sometimes I wind the lead around his legs which he doesn't like. I've so much steam to let off; I just want to run and run. I love meeting other dogs and Dad lets me say hello, but I see the other dogs running off-lead, playing and having such fun. I wish I could join in. I get home and don't feel as if I've had a walk at all. I feel very frustrated. Sometimes I find chewing the sofa helps with that, but Dad gets upset. I've also dug holes in the garden and Dad was angry I'd spoilt his flower beds. I heard him on the phone to the vet the other day. There was talk of sedatives, I do hope that's for Dad and not for me - all I want is a good run."

Active breeds need active homes

I have to admit my heart does go out to you active breeds such as Collies, Pointers, working Spaniel breeds (like myself) and Labradors, who find yourselves living in such restrictive circumstances.

Impulse buyers don't appreciate you're an active, intelligent dog with a strong working instinct, who needs a challenge. It's in your blood to use your brain.

Depending on your breed, you'll want to sniff out rabbits and pheasants, hare up a hillside herding sheep, or chase a muntjac through the woods. Your genetic make-up means you were not designed to live in a concrete urbania. Being subjected to this sort of life is for you, akin to a prison sentence. I've been told that some of you have such little stimulation in some domestic settings that you become very depressed. If you were a tortoise with a shell, no doubt you would retreat into it.

Humans who buy you on a whim don't appreciate that all you want (and need) from a walk is to be off-lead, running, sniffing, snuffling, snorting and having fun. Without this stimulation the chances are, like Ollie, you will become so frustrated and unhappy, you'll begin destroying things. Chewing the sofa, or the door frame is never popular with your humans and the repercussions will only compound your stress. Expect some very loud words to be shouted in your direction – maybe even profanities. It's possible you may be banished from human company for a while. I can only hope they don't resort to any physical retribution. At the very least they're likely to ignore you and wish you weren't there.

It's at this point that the penny may drop for the impulse-buying human and they realise their mistake. It dawns on them that they should never have brought you home in the first place. They question whether their good idea to get a dog was actually such a good idea after all.

Shouting aside, your destruction will focus their thoughts on your needs. If enough damage is done on a regular basis, not only does it make a mess, but it also affects their bank balance. Humans hate coming home after a hard day's work to a house that's been ripped asunder by your molars.

Case study: Holly the Collie

Holly the Collie found herself in a small flat, two floors up on an inner-city estate. She told Dr Peter Pointer how her home had no garden and she received no stimulation and little exercise. Holly says she soon became frustrated.

"When I was a pup, my humans played with me a lot and took me to the local playing fields with their little girl Amy. It was spring-time and I ran about and had fun. As I got bigger and stronger and the winter came, they didn't take me to the field any more. Dad was at work all day and Mum was always out doing something. I yearned for a trip to the fields and got very bored. I amused myself by chewing up some of Amy's toys. I was told off for that. I had no room to run about and nothing to do. I dreamt of rounding up sheep like my mother and grandfather had. One day, instead of Amy's toys, I began chewing the front door frame. (I thought maybe I could take myself out for a walk.) There was a lot of shouting when Dad got home. At one point I feared he was going to hit me. Not long after I chewed the door frame, I was taken

to a place with rows of kennels and lots of barking dogs. Now I'm living there too. I've not seen Mum, Dad, or Amy for a long time. I do miss them and don't know when they're coming back. The people here are very kind though and take me for a lovely walk every day."

Again, I'd never condone behaviour like Holly's, but I do sympathise and can understand the whys and wherefores. I also accept that drastic doggie circumstances call for drastic doggie action. Any sort of regular destruction is likely to lead to your human at least taking professional advice, or at worst (though it may actually be for the best), finding you a new home. It's unlikely they will have the time or inclination to change their habits to give you the fulfilled doggy life you deserve. You do run the risk of being labelled 'a dog with issues' but if that's the case, it's likely you will find a human more understanding of your needs. A new, more active home, is probably the best outcome for you.

Professor Daniel's Bones of Retention

- **Impulse buyers act on a whim**
- **You enjoy human company**
- **Your frustration isn't naughtiness**
- **You are not bad - you are bored**
- **Not all dogs want to be friends**
- **Don't bound up to dogs on leads**
- **You active breeds love brain-work**

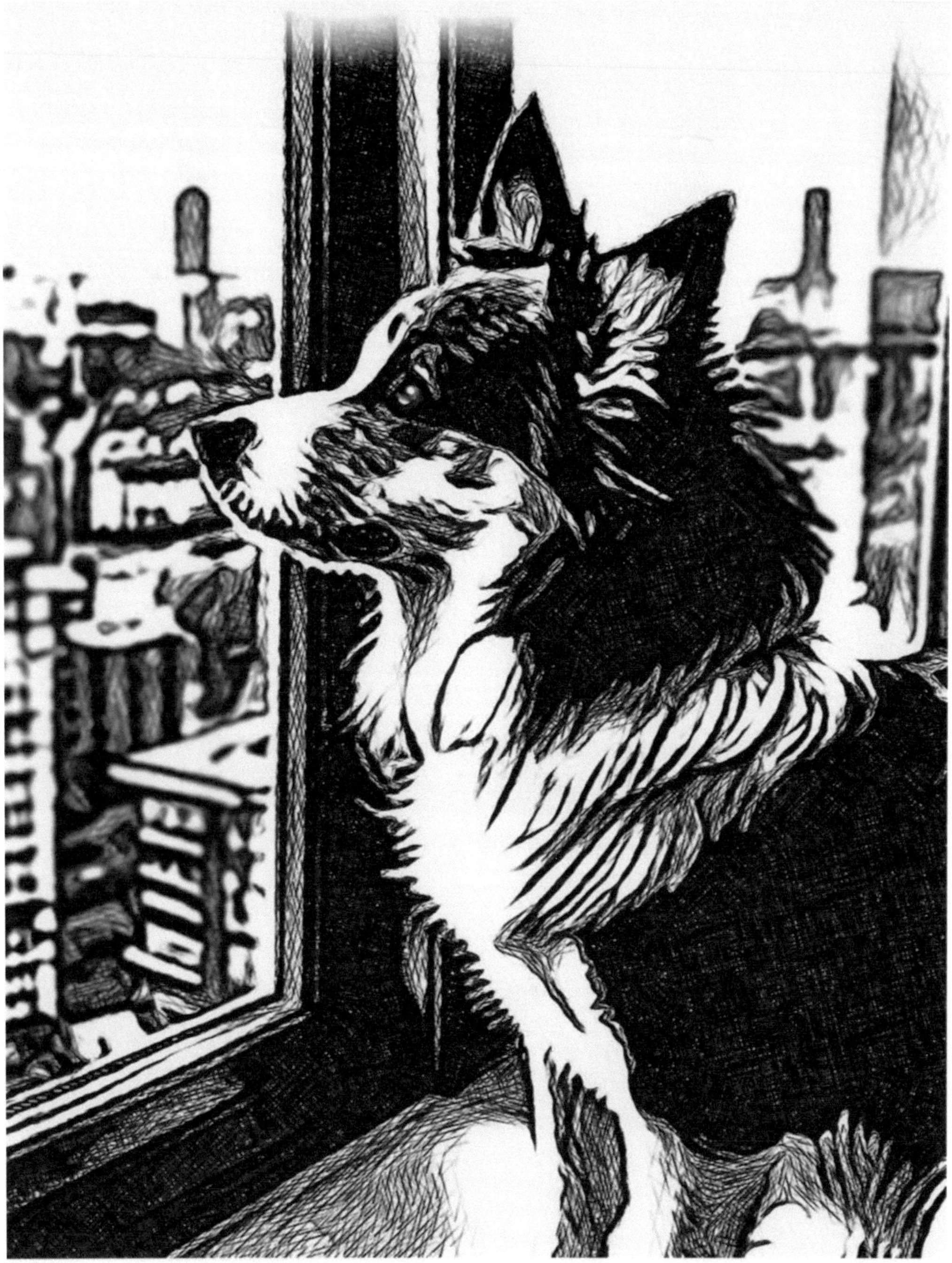

"My heart goes out to you working breeds who find yourselves in unsuitable environments."

Chapter 7

Types of humans: Best buddies

Now you may think I've been a little harsh on humans thus far. As in all walks of life you will meet humans whose position on the 'dogsense' scale will vary. For example, an impulse buyer is likely to score a 0 or 1, whereas this next type of human - your beloved best buddy, will be at the 9 or 10 level.

Those privileged pooches among you whose humans do have common sense should be very grateful. These humans will have thought things through and will go that extra mile, or even two, three, four or five for you. Before choosing you, your best buddy will have read extensively about dogs – swotting up on your characteristics and your needs. Your human will have considered long and hard which breed was best-suited to share their lifestyle, home and living location. They appreciate that having you in their home is a life-long commitment, requiring hard work, persistence, determination and dedication – to say nothing of paw-loads of patience and love.

If you're a working Collie, they know you wouldn't choose to live with them in a neat and tidy suburban semi in Slough. If you're a Working Cocker Spaniel, they sense you'll be right up their street (or more likely, down their country lane), if they're a wellie-wearing, all-weather woman in the Cotswolds. They appreciate that a more graceful (though dare I say lazier) Greyhound is perfect for a pensioner in Peterborough. If they are parents of a young family in Feckenham, they'll probably opt for an easy-going Labrador or Golden Retriever. A best buddy trail walker wanting a long-distance hiking companion, will know a Collie or hardy crossbreed fits their mountain-filled bill just perfectly. Whichever it's to be, you can bet your bottom biscuit, that your new best buddy has done their houndy-homework.

They will have checked out your breeder to ensure they were reputable (and not a puppy farmer or dog thief.) They will have met at least one of your parents and examined your family history. If you come from a family tree with dodgy hips or snappy tendencies, they will find out - and woe betide any less than honest breeder who tries pulling the fur over their eyes.

When you were about six-weeks-old, your best buddy will have picked you from your litter of siblings. (It's likely you may also have had a paw in this). After much oohing, aahing, cooing and cuddling, you were chosen for whatever traits appealed to them. Or, as if often the case, you will have chosen them. Perhaps you were the shy one who cowered quietly in the corner, the bouncy one with the biggest belly, the pushy one who was first in for a kiss, or the quietly confident one who sat and waited your turn with a knowing look in your bright blue eyes. Maybe you licked your human mum's nose, jumped on human dad's lap or weed on his or her shoe? Whatever cute tactic you employed it will have struck a strong canine chord with your starry-eyed, emotion-drunk human.

As a pup, it's easy to get humans eating out of your paws. A little hop and skip here, a lick and snuffle there. The virgin dog-owner will be well and truly smitten - and no doubt puppytooth bitten. These doey-eyed dog-lovers are now completely at your mercy. It's a hard-hearted human who isn't moved by the cuddly cuteness of you when you're a puppy.

If there is a good time to take advantage of your best buddy, this is it. Your heart-melting puppy-ness won't last forever, so do make the most of it. But remember, the best buddy type of human does have their head screwed on. They have read the books and taken sound personal advice from wise, dog-experienced friends or family. If their sensible head can keep some steadying influence over their brimming heart, they won't be swayed too much by you playing the puppy card.

You may feel they are being a 'stick-in-the-mud' (though not literally, see Chapter 10 on training) by not giving into your every whim. But believe me, they are doing you a huge, life-long favour. From day one they will apply behaviour boundaries for you. And believe me, boundaries set you up for a very happy life. From the outset, you will know where you are and what you can, or can't do. You will understand what's expected of you and what isn't. With clear house and human rules, you won't end up as a nervous wreck on anti-depressants like some of your unfortunate canine counterparts.

As a pup, your dear humans will have paid a handsome price for the honour of taking you home. Some of you will have cost thousands of their hard-earned pounds. For doggy context, I did a few sums and that equates to 1500 boxes of biscuits. Possibly more than you'll ever see in your lifetime.

You'll be parted from your siblings and your mum at between 8 - 10 weeks, which is, initially, quite unsettling. Suddenly you're on your own, with this strange-smelling human in a strange-smelling home. There will be lots of unknowns and what appear to be scary things. There will be people to investigate and you've no mum or siblings to run to for reassurance when it all gets a bit too frightening. You may feel quite alone, but this is where your feet-on-the-ground best buddy human is worth their weight in dog food.

They will know when to leave you to build up your confidence, with quiet encouragement and praise; they will know when to intervene, to prevent you hurting yourself and they will know when it's time for you to sleep, before you become over-excited and downright silly.

Some of you may be car-sick en route to your new home and you may need a wee or poo or both. Don't worry, your best buddy is prepared. They will have brought several old towels specifically for such an occurrence and won't make a fuss about it. They really do think of everything. In fact, they're as close as you'll get in a human to being almost as clever as we are.

Once in your new home, a veritable room-full of comfort and fun awaits you. You'll be provided with a cosy bed or crate with access to a wipe-clean floor. You'll have a number of squeaking and soft toys to entertain you and something warm and snuggly to cuddle up with at bedtime.

If you're very lucky, your human breeder may have packed you off with a little blanket that holds the scent of your doggy mum. If there are other animals in the household, your human will be very cautious when introducing you. It's likely they will do this on neutral territory at first, so older canines in the family don't feel too protective of their home and humans. They'll also ensure you don't get spat at, or your cornea scratched out on your first day by one of those haughty, hissy felines. None of us want to go through life with one eye, a torn ear or scarred cheek.

Your best buddy human won't expose you to potentially life-threatening doggy viruses before you are fully vaccinated. Any trips out will be confined to the car or their arms. Once you're fully protected from the health threats of the outside world, your socialisation and training will begin with them in earnest.

If you're lucky enough to have landed in the home of a best buddy, you really have landed on your paws. They are prepared, knowledgeable and ready to put in the time, training and to be honest, the darned hard work it takes to bring up a pup. They will be consistent with commands, loving and kind (of course), firm but fair (necessary) and lavish you with praise and love when you do what's asked of you.

Case study: Polly the Poodle

Polly was 9-weeks-old when her human family of best buddies, took her home. She's now six months-old. She tells Dr Peter Pointer about her early days.

"My first night was strange. I was on my own in a metal crate. I was a bit scared and I whined and cried for my mum. I hoped someone would come, but no one did. My bed was warm and cosy so I eventually drifted off to sleep. I grew to love my crate; it's my cosy safe place. Mum put me in it regularly for sleep-time when I was very little. I had three meals a day and was taken outside regularly so I could do my business. Mum watched me like a hawk. I soon learned to stand at the door when I needed a wee or poo. Now I'm a bit bigger, I can hold it much longer. I'm not allowed upstairs or on the sofa, but I have my own chair with a snuggly

blanket I can sit on. I also have my own comfy bed and my crate. I've learned to come when I'm called, to walk to heel and not pull on the lead. I get lots of walks in the countryside where I run about off the lead, exploring. I get lots of fuss and cuddles and playtime in the garden with toys and games. I love my human family. I know exactly what's expected of me and I know that if I do what's asked of me, I get even more praise and treats."

If you're what humans call a rescue dog, you'll need a slight variation - a special human known as a 'best-ever buddy'. That's one who does their very best AND has experience of supporting troubled doggy souls.

You may be adopted from a rescue centre or have arrived from abroad – like our friends from countries such as Romania, Ireland and Greece. Some of you are rehomed privately by impulse buyers who realise their mistake once you are around 12 months old.

If you're a rescued or rehomed dog, your best-ever buddy, will try to find out as much as possible about your past. You could be mistaken for thinking you're in a 'Which Doggy Do You Think You Are? programme. But fear not, your investigative human is simply finding out all they can about your breed and how they can most help you. Beware, if you're related to a canine with a dubious background (criminal, unknown, or unreliable parentage), your Sherlock Human may well unearth it and will want to know all about that too.

They may send your DNA to a lab for testing. (That's not to a Labrador, but a laboratory). They'll discover what percentage of which breeds you are. Though it makes not a sniff of difference to you, it helps them identify any specific likes or dislikes, tendencies or traits you may display. For instance, Belgian Malinois are natural protectors, Dachshunds have long, vulnerable backs, Whippets (and Greyhounds) dislike the cold and wet, Poodles have a propensity to be anxious.

If out of the blue, you are suddenly taken on a 10-mile craggy hill run, it's probably because your DNA shows you are 60 per cent Trailhound. If you are dragged unhappily up a snow-capped mountain, it may be your make-up is largely St Bernard or Burmese Mountain Dog. If you are unexpectedly invited to catch rats in a farmer's barn, consider yourself of strong Terrier extraction. Though given the choice, you may prefer to stay curled up by the fire, thank you very much.

Your best-ever buddy will also learn of your less-endearing qualities. But fear not, they will not judge you. Maybe you hate joggers, or want to chase cars and cyclists? (Common Collie traits.) Are you a sheep-chaser or child-nipper? (Let's be honest, we've all wanted to at some point.) Are you frightened of old men in caps, or do you shake if you see a woman with a stick?

Such behaviour won't deter your best-ever buddy. In fact, they will do all they can to support and reassure you. What are perceived as bad traits by some less robust humans, do not deter these pillars of doggy society. They are endowed with kennels full of human kindness and understand these behaviours are not your fault. They appreciate most aggressive behaviour is more often than not, the result of deep-seated fears, in most cases caused by the actions of the final type of humans known as bad beings. (More on those in the following chapter.)

Case study: Lottie the Labrador

Lottie is a former gun dog and good friend of Dr Peter Pointer. He helped her settle into domestic life with a best-ever buddy and come to terms with some of the trauma of her early years.

"I spent my first three years being trained to be a gun dog by a man with a heavy hand and an even heavier boot. I was pulled and kicked, this way and that. One day he hauled me up by the scruff of my neck for the umpteenth time, shouting and swearing into my face. I was so terrified that I bit him. Later that day, I was delivered - without even a collar or lead - to a local rescue centre. I was rehomed to a kind family but when some male relatives visited, I bit them. I was returned to the rescue centre where a male kennel worker tried to coax me out of bed by the collar. I was so scared, I bit him too. One day a woman visited me. She talked to me gently and sat with me on the floor. She stroked me slowly and calmly. For the first time in years, I stretched out on my side and nearly relaxed. This woman visited me lots of times and brought me bits of sausage. One day she took me home. It was all new and I was pretty terrified. I just sat, curled up tightly, flinching at the slightest sound or movement she made. The one good thing was that there were no men in the house. My new mum let me do things at my own pace and in my own time. She never forced me to do anything I didn't want to, or to go anywhere that frightened me. She never raised her voice to me. She sat quietly and massaged me and bit by bit, I felt my nervous tension melting away. At first, I wasn't happy around other dogs, so my new mum insisted I wore a muzzle. She took me up hills, in woods, to the seaside and I had my own quiet field where I learnt to be a dog without fear. I feel so

different now. I'm no longer scared of men and greet them happily for fuss. I don't wear a muzzle anymore and socialise with other dogs. I didn't realise my life could be so happy and full of love. I'm still a bit anxious of sudden noises or quick movements. I instantly cower as they trigger memories of my old life. But I know Mum is always here for me with her love and understanding. I know I'm safe now and I'll never be hurt again."

Although Lottie's first rehoming didn't work out, she did find her forever home. Her story shows you should never give up hope if you find yourself in a similar situation. There are always best-ever buddies out there.

Some of you may have been bought as pups during the human world's Covid-19 pandemic. Many of them became very ill during this period and everyone had to stay at home. It was also a time when many humans who'd never owned dogs before, bought their first puppies. Of course, as a cuddly bundle with a black button nose and sweet-scented fur, you were irresistible. But you grew larger and bouncier. Often untrained and unruly, you found yourself at the doors of local animal shelters.

Then came the human world's cost-of-living crisis. With soaring expenses, some families simply couldn't afford to keep you any longer. The result? Rescue centres are full of dogs needing homes and animal charities are under immense pressure.

There are occasions when you may be rehomed to unsuitable humans. Love seekers and impulse buyers can be very good at convincing shelters they would make perfect pet parents. Sometimes they'll tell outright porky pies about their

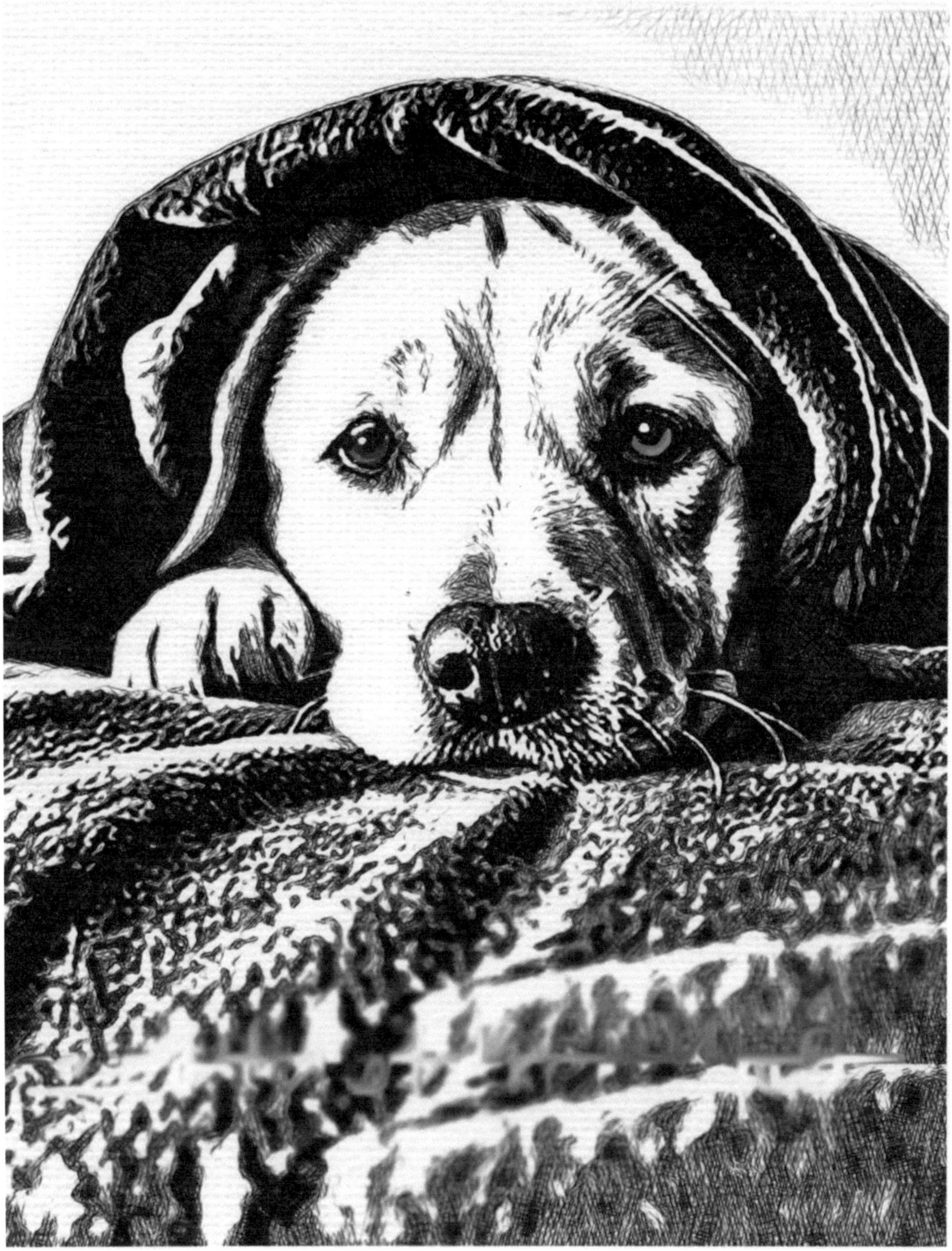

"If you're in the home of a best buddy you really have landed on your paws."

living or working arrangements to meet the charity's rehoming criteria.

In reality, these humans simply want their own way and expect you to fit into their lives. What they don't realise is, that many rescue dogs with traumatic histories, cannot easily fit in. If this proves to be the case, sadly, days, weeks or months later, you may be returned with your tail between your legs and a tear in your eye – having endured an uncomfortable period, not living up to your adopter's expectations.

Don't worry, with a bit of Lassie luck a best-ever buddy will be along to find you and, as in Lottie's case, you'll receive all the support, understanding, time, patience and love that you deserve.

Professor Daniel's Bones of Retention

- **Best buddies know about your breed**
- **Make the most of being a cute puppy**
- **Best-ever buddies go the extra mile**
- **Puppies cost at least 1500 boxes of biscuits**
- **Your best buddy nearly always knows best**
- **Best buddies have paw-loads of patience**
- **Best buddies are nearly as clever as you**

Chapter 8

Types of humans: Bad beings

I won't devote much space (or time) to the final type of human, the 'bad being". This is because, in my view they don't deserve it. I'm even uncomfortable calling them humans, as I feel it's an insult to all your good, kind and decent human parents. At first glance, these beings are perceived as humans. They walk, talk, look and appear like any other dog-owner, but there are one or two major differences. Their hearts are as hard as stone and their emotions as cold as ice.

As sensitive souls, you know instinctively these are not good people to be around. Bad beings view dogs as mere things. Things to be used, abused and exploited. Either for their financial gain, employment or enjoyment. However, should your performance wane, your usefulness ebb or you don't make the grade, you will be discarded like a wrung-out dishcloth, without a moment's thought. You are no longer viable, or of any financial worth to these beings.

In reality you may be only two or three-years-old. Even in dog years that's no age at all and paws crossed, you still have a lot of life left to live. But if you were a racing, breeding, shooting or trailing dog, you may find yourself out on your well-clipped ear, before you're even three-years-old.

Don't expect any thanks or appreciation for your loyalty, hard work and hours of tireless effort. On the contrary, your early dismissal will have you labelled as useless, past your best, or simply no good.

Once your talent for racing, breeding or working declines, a bad being won't want you cluttering up their kennels if you aren't earning your keep. When this happens, some of you will be sent, or a better word might be dumped, at a rescue centre with not so much as a backward glance. Consider yourself privileged to end up there, for there are those who aren't so lucky – and they won't be reading this.

I've heard spine-chilling stories from some of you who were racers, trailers, breeders and retrievers. You've told of the hardships, cruelty and evils you endured at the hands of these bad beings. With no way out and nowhere to turn, the only place left for you to go is inwards. You shut yourselves down. I've met dogs who became frozen, petrified, empty shells. Too frightened and traumatised to feel or function. Overworked, overpowered and overwhelmed. Their natural doggie spirit, for which we're so famed and adored, had completely evaporated, like steam from a canine kettle.

To me it's quite obvious that a dog won't thrive on dominating, or controlling behaviour. Many of these bad beings have huge egos and no compassion. Now, egos are not part of your psyche, but sadly, they are very much apparent in humans. Egos are often the bane of your lives, responsible for much pain, suffering, violence and hatred.

I've talked to canine colleagues who were starved, beaten, tied up, kicked and forced into cages. Some who were locked in laboratories to be used in experiments. Others who were kept prisoner in dark, dank sheds and forced to breed over and over again.

Others of you were bred only to race, run, or retrieve, trained by aggressive bullies with stick-wielding hands and hefty boots. This isn't a life, it's an existence and a miserable one at that. No tasty treats, affection or fur-roasting fireside for you. It makes me incredibly sad for to think of those of you who are enduring, or have been subjected to such cruelty.

Case study: Tessie the Trailhound

Tessie was bred to race over the fells in the north of England. She told Dr Peter Pointer that she didn't make the grade and as a result suffered at the hands of a bad being.

"I was the runt of the litter, much smaller than my siblings and not considered strong enough to race. I was taken away from my family when I was young. I was left alone in a dark, damp stone building. A man in a cap and big coat would come in. He'd regularly pick me up by the scruff of the neck and shake me, often shouting too. When he'd finished venting his anger on me, I was dropped to the floor. Once he threw me against the wall. I don't know what I'd done wrong but I was terrified of him. I missed my mum and siblings terribly and I felt very sad and lonely. When I was about 12-months-old, a woman came to the shed. She drove me to a place full of other dogs known as a rescue centre. I was first rehomed to a man, but I was so scared of him, I cowered in a corner for a week and wouldn't go near him so I was soon back at the centre. Then my luck changed. Two women saw me hiding at the back of my kennel and realised how scared I was. One of them took me home. I had never lived in a house before so was frightened of everything. I jumped on the table and climbed on the window ledges. For a long time, I weed and pooed on the floor.

Even then, my human mum didn't give up on me – despite me chewing the door frame. Being a Trailhound, I was bred to run, so she took me jogging and I loved that; it helped me to relax. My new mum showed me that not all humans are cruel. She showed me love, patience and understanding. It took me years before I stopped cowering in fright from men in caps. With her love and support I grew more confident, fun-loving and carefree. I now have a very happy life with my human mum."

Bad beings are devoid of feelings

I believe bad beings are devoid of any emotional intelligence – in stark contrast to you and to our lovely best buddy humans. Your naturally compassionate and caring natures mean you possess this in abundance. These bad beings are the worst types of humans that you, as sensitive doggie souls, could have the misfortune to meet and I sincerely hope you never do.

For those of you who are experiencing, or have been subjected to these unfeeling monsters, my heart goes out to you. You may well find yourself in a fear-driven fight for survival. Your only remaining defence (and the last resort) if you have the strength of spirit, is to bite. Whether it be their hands, feet, ankles or legs. However, I know that if you do, the repercussions from a bad being are severe.

This is one instance when I would advocate running away if you possibly can. Flee as far as you can safely go. With four sound paws and a sensitive snout, you may be lucky and wise enough to sniff out some safe haven. If you're picked up on the street as a stray, you will probably end up at a rescue centre. If so, it will be full of kind-hearted people, more best buddy types of humans who will help find you a home with another of their kind. It may take some time, but at least you will be safe, loved, well-looked after and, more importantly, no longer used and abused, physically and emotionally.

Trauma as a youngster can affect you forever

Even with the love and kindness of a best-ever buddy, some of you may never recover fully from the traumatic experiences you suffered at the hands of a bad being. This is something we do have in common with humans. If they suffer sustained mental and physical abuse over a prolonged period, especially when they're young, it takes a huge toll on them too. Neither dogs, nor people come out of these cruel experiences unscathed.

Many of you will carry these emotional scars to lesser or greater doggy degrees, for the rest of your lives. You will need special humans to help you through it. Human adults and children are much the same. For many of you, these dark days lurk like a bad smell in your memory, resurfacing when you least expect it. Trauma often becomes deeply embedded in your physical body and can manifest as illness, behavioural issues, or both.

Best-ever buddies understand you've had a very hard and unhappy life and will make huge allowances for you. But they may not always appreciate just how traumatic life was for you, or how deeply it affected you. If they watch your body language however, they will see the mental and physical scars you carry.

Always remember - you are a survivor. It's in your make-up to be forever optimistic and loyal, always hoping the next human to cross your path will be better. (Let's face it, they could hardly be any worse.) So, being a stoic, uncomplaining canine, you will soldier bravely on, whatever life, or a bad being, throws at you. Your spirit may be dulled with sadness and your body pained from stress, but once you're free from these tyrannical types, I promise you, your life will improve greatly.

Repairing your damage will take time

God-willing, you'll end up in much kinder hands – ideally those of a best-ever buddy. They are naturally loving and caring. They will do all they can to help you overcome your anxieties, build your confidence and help you move on. Given time, love, patience and the right support in the right home with the right human, you will find life worth living again. Always remember, you are a highly sensitive being. You are not a broken machine, that with the addition of a new part can be quickly repaired. Your 'repair' will take longer. Depending on your history, it may be several years before your fears fade. Some of you will find those fears never leave you entirely. The effects of deep-seated and sustained trauma will sit heavily within you, but I promise you - they can be released.

Once you are free from the tyrant that is a bad being, you'll face the challenge of adapting and adjusting to a new life. Don't expect this to happen overnight, or even in a few days, weeks or months for that matter. It's unlikely you will become the happy, bouncy dog you were born to be, in such a short period of time.

Even with a kind and loving best-ever buddy, your years of abuse may weigh heavily on your shaky shoulders. Your new human would no more kick or hit you than eat your dinner, but don't be surprised if you find yourself cowering when your new owner approaches. You may even find yourself, against your better judgement, reacting aggressively if asked to do something that scares you. You may snap or even attempt to bite, if someone tries to put you in a car, or fit you with a collar or harness. It's not that you are an aggressive dog, far from it. It's because your brain is hard-wired to react like this. You do it instinctively, for your own protection, it's your survival mechanism.

Case study: Beauty the Beagle

Beauty's story is anything but pretty. She was bred for experiments in a laboratory. Dr Peter Pointer is well-acquainted with her history and is helping her adapt to life outside the lab. This is what she told him.

"It was an extremely unhappy and distressing place to live. We were kept in large wire cages and were never taken out. We had no stimulation. As a result, many dogs barked a lot and repeatedly ran or paced back and forth. Sometimes I was taken into a laboratory that smelt of chemicals. Men took blood from my ear and sometimes my teeth were taken out. I heard from other dogs that they were feeding us high levels of sugar and then testing us to monitor the impact on our bodies. It all became too much for me. One day I just threw myself at a wall. If any men came near, I would try to bite them and squealed if they touched my ears. I began eating my poo. Looking back, I think I was having a nervous breakdown. I couldn't cope any longer and just shut down. It was after this that I was taken to a dog rescue centre. I find it hard to trust humans now. I was rehomed to a lovely couple and life is

much better, but I still feel very sad. I've yet to feel carefree and happy as I know other dogs do."

Kind homes and happy times await you

If you've been subjected to years of physical or emotional abuse, you become conditioned to react like this. With time, patience, understanding and love from your best-ever buddy you will get used to your new life of love. It may take you several years to adjust, but once you relax into a cruelty-free life full of compassion, your tail will wag forever. (See Chapter 12 where I talk more about your mental health and available help.)

My research shows that once your traumatic past has been acknowledged by your new human, it's better for you if they don't dwell on those dark and dismal times. It does you no good to be reminded of the fearful life you previously led. Your former life carries a negativity and sadness with it. It's a dense feeling that, as far as you're concerned, is best left in the past. Hearing your human talk of your dark days isn't healthy for you. You'll feel as if you're being followed around by a heavy, gloomy cloud. Such repeated reminders make it harder for your blue skies and sunshine to emerge. What's done is done.

Your life now is one of happiness and love. Your future is full of hope, and that's all that's important for you now. Strive to live as you were meant to, and as only dogs can. Enjoy every day and seize every moment with excitement and gusto.

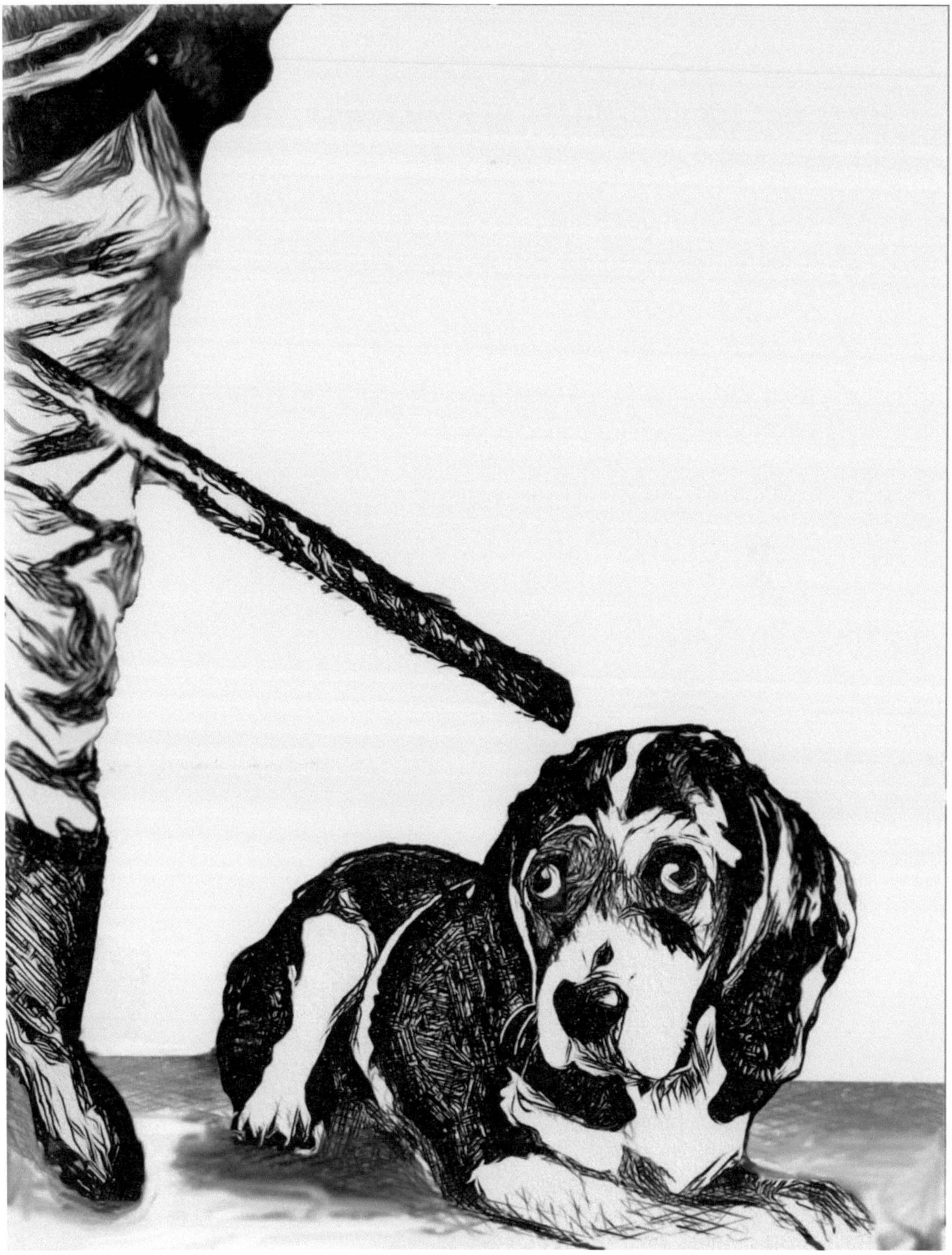

"You won't thrive on dominating and controlling behaviour. Bad beings have no compassion."

Professor Daniel's Bones of Retention

- Bad beings have hearts of stone
- You are not a 'thing'
- Rescue centres are full of best buddies
- You are a survivor
- Cruelty can be overcome
- Give yourself time to adjust (think years, not months)
- Love and support await you

Chapter 9

Boundaries: Being your best or worst selves

When your human welcomes you as a cuddly pup into their home, their hearts and arms are wide open. However, this means there is one important thing they may overlook - setting you some healthy boundaries.

Now by boundaries, I mean making it clear to you what behaviour you can or cannot get away with. Think of them as your doggy principles, what's acceptable or unacceptable as far as you and your human are concerned. It's a sort of doggy etiquette, the unwritten understanding between you both.

Cricket, a traditional English game played by humans, provides a good visual example. The ground on which the match is played has boundaries, lines that if the ball or players cross, certain rules are enforced. Boundaries with you and your human are no different. There are invisible lines, or codes of canine conduct, that are made clear and mustn't be crossed.

For example, your human may set a boundary such as, they don't want you licking their face. If you try to do this you will likely hear a firm "no," and be gently pushed away. Your human makes it obvious your behaviour on the face-licking front is not acceptable to them.

Many humans will disapprove of you helping yourself to mouth-watering meals that they've left on the side. There may be drool-inducing aromas wafting around your head and your belly may be gurgling like an old drain, but the boundary is set and it's more than your year's supply of biscuits is worth, to as much as raise your snout to that steaming plate of steak.

Similarly, if you help yourself to that temptingly discarded rind of tasty cheddar on a plate on the coffee table, you cross the 'don't steal food' boundary and a firm scolding may ensue.

If you're a pushy Pug pup with an appetite of a pig, your human will need to adopt a very robust approach. They will need to set a firm boundary in response to your repeated whines and whinges for an extra treat or titbit. They may be tempted to give in to your daily demands for the latest delicacy because you look so sweet. But if they succumb to your pitiful pleadings, you risk ending up as a pretty podgy (and unhealthy) pooch, who spends much of their time under everyone's feet snuffling for snacks.

Human hearts can rule their heads

Now your squidgy-hearted humans are, of course, staring gooey-eyed at you through their rose-tinted, puppy-focused spectacles. This means that at this stage, any semblance of sense is in danger of going straight out of their doggy-drunk little heads. But if your human has the presence and strength of mind to say no when required, you will grow up the better dog for it. Allowing their hearts to rule their heads means you'll have no boundaries in your human-canine relationship and, as with training, it can result in some real doggy dilemmas as you grow up.

Case study: Gracie the Great Dane

Gracie was bought from a reputable breeder by her human family and taken home at 9-weeks-old. As a pup she was the centre of their world. As she grew bigger, she told Dr Peter Pointer she always seemed to be in trouble.

"When I was a pup, everything I did made my humans laugh. I was allowed to sit on the sofa with the children for cuddles and potter about in the kitchen when Mum was cooking. She would give me little bits of food she was preparing. Sometimes the children would carry me upstairs to lie on the bed with them when their parents weren't looking. As I grew into an adult dog, I carried on doing the same things, but nobody laughed anymore. Mum would shout at me, saying I was in her way and being a nuisance. Once she fell over me and twisted her ankle. I was shut in the utility room for a while after that. When I try to get on the sofa with the children for cuddles, they shout and cry saying I'm too big and heavy and that I hurt them. I then get really told off by Mum or Dad. I seem to be in trouble most of the time. I don't understand why they're not laughing now; I'm not doing anything different."

For your human's part they need to protect and respect your boundaries too. If you're clearly uncomfortable in certain situations or with some people, I would hope your human appreciates and supports your feelings. Ideally this means not forcing you into situations in which you are obviously unhappy or frightened. This boundary business works both ways.

Now I know that as a pup you will find it great fun to explore where you want, when you want and do what you want. But, take it from me, your canine character is not suited to this

1960s-style free-for-all. It certainly won't bring your humans any 'peace man' and it doesn't allow anyone, including you, to 'just chill'.

In this respect, you're much like children. You're so much happier (and better behaved), when you know where you stand (or sit, play, sleep, run and toilet), though hopefully not all in the same place!

You may recall your biological mum assumed this role as soon as you were born. She was your 'doggy maitre'd' - the undisputed mistress of the house. The house, in your case being a large bed, or a small pen that kept her piglet-like litter (yes that's you) safely secure.

From the minute you arrived into the world, blind and squeaking, you were kept in line by your mum. Mums are great. They know all about doggy etiquette, humans and you. Your mum always has the upper paw and it can be a very strong one at that. As you grow bigger and bolder, you must abide by her rules until you are taken from her cosy and secure care.

Demand too much attention, or be too pushy over food and you can expect a rebuking, maternal nip. Put yourself and your siblings in danger and you'll be speedily scooped up in her gentle jaws and carried squirming and helpless to safety.

As you grow, play and explore with your siblings, she will watch out for and keep in check any errant behaviour on your part. Overstepping of any canine marks will be addressed immediately, without fuss. Severe maternal reprimands may involve a low growl, or curling of lips. You'll be well-advised to take note and do as you are warned.

If your canine mum continued to oversee you, her natural and instinctive boundaries would serve as an excellent doggy rule book for you. In reality, this doesn't happen often. You are left to the devices (some good, some bad, some non-existent) of your new human.

Now to my mind, this is when your human needs to step up to the doggy plate (NB: It will be empty because no self-respecting dog has a full plate.) She needs to take over the 'canine mum' mantle and keep you on the straight and narrow, behaviour-wise. Ideally, your new human will have learnt through either reading, doing online research, talking to a trainer or to wise, dog-owning friends, that healthy boundaries are one of the most vital components they need to follow during your puppyhood and beyond.

Beware an almighty all-paws fall

Without them, your future happiness and mental health are likely to go one way and one way only - down the doggy drain. If you live with a human who sets you no healthy behaviour boundaries, they are setting you (and themselves) up for an almighty, all-paws fall.

Sadly, I see and hear the results of this major oversight all too often. Much heartache, headache and an unruly and even damaged home will surely follow. Your human will notice visitors staying away and humans getting physically injured – and all because you grew up in a home that was little more than an undisciplined doggy den of iniquity.

Now I believe some humans find it difficult to set boundaries because in truth, they are not entirely content souls themselves. There is a degree of co-dependency in the mix, so having healthy boundaries is a most difficult business. You're at risk of ruling their lives as they pander to your every whim, but this isn't good for your houndy health. You're likely to grow into a very demanding, needy dog who cannot stand on its own four paws. You probably won't be comfortable if you're left alone and may be fearful in the presence of other canines.

Love-seeking humans do enjoy and crave your attention. They find it easier to give in to your emotional demands, than to consistently uphold a firm "no." In their slightly strange, human heads, they fear that if they don't allow you to do what you want, you will stop loving them. They will feel bad or mean. These are not words to which we canines attach any meaning, but humans excel at judgement, especially of themselves as far as you're concerned. This is why they repeatedly give in to any doleful-eyed look you care to throw their way.

Now the idea we would stop loving them is a ridiculous notion. It's one only a human could dream up. We all know you love unconditionally and loyally; that's what you do. It would take more than an insistent "get down", or "no", to stop you loving your human. Even those poor doggy souls who are cruelly treated, still show loyalty to their human. But as my Grandmother Gertie always said, "there's no fool like a human fool."

You're a vision of complete cuddliness

You'll learn that humans can be easily taken in, especially when you're young. They see you only as loveliness on four legs. It's absolutely true - of course you are. You're a veritable vision of complete cuddliness. No disputing that. Who wouldn't be bowled over by you - an enthusiastic, cute, innocent, new furry friend? But these humans can let their emotions completely overrule any common sense they may have. And as I've said before, a lot of humans have little common sense – even less so when it comes to you.

As an incredibly lovable puppy, you can get away with almost anything. A little snuffle here, or lick there and you'll have your human wrapped around your tiny, paddy paws. (Especially if they are impulse buyers, or love seekers.) A best buddy is aware of this dangerous pitfall and will do their utmost to stick to their boundaries. It may sound a little harsh, but believe me, it's not. They are kind, loving and caring humans who want the best for you in the long term. If they give in to your bright, pleading eyes now, they know it won't do you (them, or anyone else for that matter) any furry favours further down the doggy line.

Unfortunately, if you live with an impulse buyer or a love seeker, you could be in for a confusing time. Without healthy boundaries, you will have complete doggy freedom to do as you please. You'll be playing and biting as roughly as you want, running where you like, when you like, jumping up on whoever you fancy, demanding attention at the drop of a biscuit and basically doing your own thing, both in and outside the home.

I've learnt that a human can have quite a battle on their hands (or more to the point in their heads) when trying to take a firm emotional stance with you. Now let's be honest, whether you're an adoringly cute pup, or a delectable fully-grown dog, you really can turn on the canine charm if you want something badly enough. It's when their hearts are melted by those magical moments that your human runs the risk of letting those boundaries slip.

You may be labelled a mad, bad, naughty dog

As you grow – and depending on your breed – I can assure you that the novelty of your unchecked puppy behaviour without boundaries, will wear thin, along with your human's patience. Once you grow into a sturdy young dog, your human will suddenly expect you to do as you're told. They will wonder why you keep jumping up at them. They can't understand why you pester and bark at them and cause mayhem if left alone.

It's likely that some of these humans will blame you. They will describe you as a bad dog, a mad dog or a naughty dog. They will complain to family and friends that you are uncontrollable, that you won't do as you're told and are ruining their personal relationships, or even their lives. There may be talk of rehoming you.

They could find that family and friends no longer want to visit. It's hardly surprising. No human wants to be nipped or scratched, have their glasses broken and their handbag strap chewed, on what should be a pleasant Sunday afternoon gathering. I know pinching glasses and chewing bags and shoes is fun and a popular soother if you're teething, but humans won't be impressed.

Humans often lay the blame at your paws, when it's actually their lack of clear boundaries that has put you both in this unacceptable and untenable situation. If truth be told, you aren't really happy or relaxed living this hectic, lawless existence and your human most certainly isn't.

Your impulse buyers and love seekers may be under the mistaken illusion that once you grow up, you will magically transform (Labracadabrador-like) into a well-behaved adult dog. I'm not sure how many magic shows they've attended, but I've yet to see this happen myself.

Pups are like children. When young they need constant guidance, clear rules of what behaviour is and isn't acceptable and for it to be stated consistently and calmly over and over again. If they had a broken record and a turntable player, it would be well-worth their time putting on the vinyl entitled 'Boundaries' by the singer 'One Sensible Human' and listening to it on repeat.

During the boundary setting sessions, should your human get stressed, raise their voice, or God forbid, physically hit out at you in frustration, this does nothing to achieve your end good dog goal.

You need time and hard work from your human

Some humans, and there are sadly quite a lot of them, do not realise how much time and hard work is required to ensure you grow into a secure, rounded (but not in the belly department) dog. It's a sad but true fact, that many humans do not possess the time, patience, temperament or understanding to set and abide by doggy boundaries.

An added confusion factor for you, is if several humans in the household are nurturing you. To be your best doggy self, everyone needs to stick together. To howl off the same hymn sheet, if you will. This will not work if, despite your human mum or dad setting clear boundaries, you're given the opposite message by a younger, or older, household member. If third parties disregard your human's doggy house rules, you will be left utterly discom-dogulated.

Others in the family may find it amusing to flaunt your rules, but they don't realise how very confusing this is for you. On one hand you have your human dad sternly saying you're not allowed in the bedroom. Then one evening, with the backs of parents turned, Daisy the teenager daughter carries you triumphantly upstairs to her bedroom. Similarly, when generous Granny comes to visit, you're encouraged to hop up onto her lap on the comfy, soft sofa – somewhere your mum has decreed, in no uncertain terms, is definitely out of bounds for those paddy puppy paws.

This leaves you with no idea where you sit or stand, whether you should be up, down, on or off the stairs. You'll get cuddles and fuss for going upstairs with daughter Daisy, but a scary, scolding voice from a most disapproving dad. That would leave even the brightest of you not knowing which way to wag for the best.

Talking of fuss and cuddles, one of your human's greatest pitfalls is thinking they should give you constant attention. They shouldn't. Of course, you enjoy it, who doesn't? You will lap it up. But you don't need it constantly. Humans are outrageously bad at setting boundaries in this area. Ensuring you respect each other's personal space is imperative to a happy human and dog relationship.

You shouldn't have the upper paw

Think back to your doggy mum. If you were constantly in her face and bothering her, she would get up and walk away. If you persist in your eager, puppy-like way, you may even receive a warning 'back off' nip, or a growl to tell you to do as you're told. I'm not saying your human should nip you (though I have heard of some old shepherds nipping their dogs' ears if they did something wrong.) But for your sake, humans should adhere to personal space boundaries. In reality, this means not allowing you the upper paw so you won't constantly make a nuisance of yourself.

I know many humans find this incredibly challenging. It's as if they have an 'obliged to respond to the dog' switch in their heads. One look or nudge from you and they're at your beck and call, fawning around like some love-sick teenager. With clear boundaries, you can both sit happily and quietly in your own spaces, settled and at peace.

This doesn't mean you don't love each other. Of course not. It means your bond is strong enough that neither needs constant reassurance from the other. Likewise, you will each enjoy having a corner to call your own. If you are brought up with boundaries, you soon learn you don't always have to be the centre of attention. You will contentedly snooze in your own space, resting and digesting as balanced dogs should. If not, you're likely to be jumping up at anyone who as much as breathes in your direction. This will annoy the hell out of your humans and I can't say I blame them.

Case study: Zippit the Whippet

Zippit, also known as Zippy, lived with a young couple who rehomed him from a rescue centre. He was the centre of their life – then a baby came along. Here, he tells Dr Peter Pointer what happened.

"I was so lucky to find my humans and they doted on me. If I wanted to curl up in between them on the sofa when they were cuddling, I could. Mum always let me lie under the bed covers with them too, even though Dad wasn't happy about that. One day I noticed Mum's stomach was growing and I sensed something was happening. There was a feeling of excitement, concern and anticipation from Mum and lots of decorating being done by Dad. One night they disappeared and I was left alone. I didn't like that and began chewing up their duvet. Dad told me off very sternly when he got back. When Mum came home a few days later, she had a tiny human in a carrycot. I didn't much like the look of it. It was the focus of everyone's attention. Nobody was cuddling or talking to me anymore. I began whining and barking to get their attention. Mum and Dad didn't like me doing that as it woke up the tiny human and it started crying too. I tried climbing up on Mum's lap like I used to, but she had this tiny human held close to her and pushed me away. I wasn't happy about that so began barking at her. I leapt up on the back of the sofa and lay down there instead. Dad saw what happened and got very cross with me. He tried to pull me off the sofa away from Mum so I bit him. They seem to have forgotten how they always give me everything I want."

Having time out to snooze quietly and uninterrupted is one of the healthiest habits your human can help you to develop. Without it, your bombarded doggy brain becomes scrambled. You will end up literally chasing your tail. It's just as important for your human to rest and digest too (but that's a whole different book). If you can do it together, what a contented picture of domestic doggy bliss that makes.

Even you small breeds are still dogs at heart

If you are a small breed such as a Dachshund, Shih Tzu, or Chihuahua, the setting of boundaries comes with an added layer of confusion. I call it the 'itsy bitsy' boundary. Due to your diminutive dimensions, impulse buyers and love seekers are likely to be very protective of you. They will pick you up at every opportunity and carry you around.

On the outside, you may enjoy this type of sedan-chair treatment. You could be forgiven for thinking yourself some sort of canine king or queen. But – and this is a pretty big dog-defying but – it means you don't get to behave, or live, like the dog you really are.

The best thing your human can do with you if you're a small breed, is to let you be a dog. Just because you are closer to the ground, doesn't make you any less of a canine. You still want to sniff, run, play, socialise and explore. Being treated as some lesser Lassie who needs to be constantly in your human's arms, is one of the worst types of doggy mollycoddling.

It's the blurring of boundaries in true HuDog fashion. You're likely to grow up with irrational reactions. Barking and cowering in fear whenever your tiny feet do get to touch the ground, or snarling at perceived threats, if ever you are allowed to walk at your rightful, lower level.

If you have no itsy bitsy boundaries, you won't feel comfortable in your own little skin. Your human has made the common mistake of thinking they are protecting you. It is indeed their love and concern for you that drives this, which is admirable of course. But sadly, it won't help you grow into a balanced dog.

Being a pup in a human world can be challenging enough at the best of times. It requires clear boundaries applied consistently, patiently and with understanding. This is quite the list for your human to follow and to successfully achieve it over many months is a tall order – whether you've got short legs or not.

Professor Daniel's Bones of Retention:

- **Boundaries give you peace of mind**
- **Some humans can't say no**
- **Get used to your own company**
- **Whatever your size, you are still a dog**
- **Abide by your human's house rules**
- **Some humans lead you astray**
- **Bad doggie behaviour is rarely your fault**

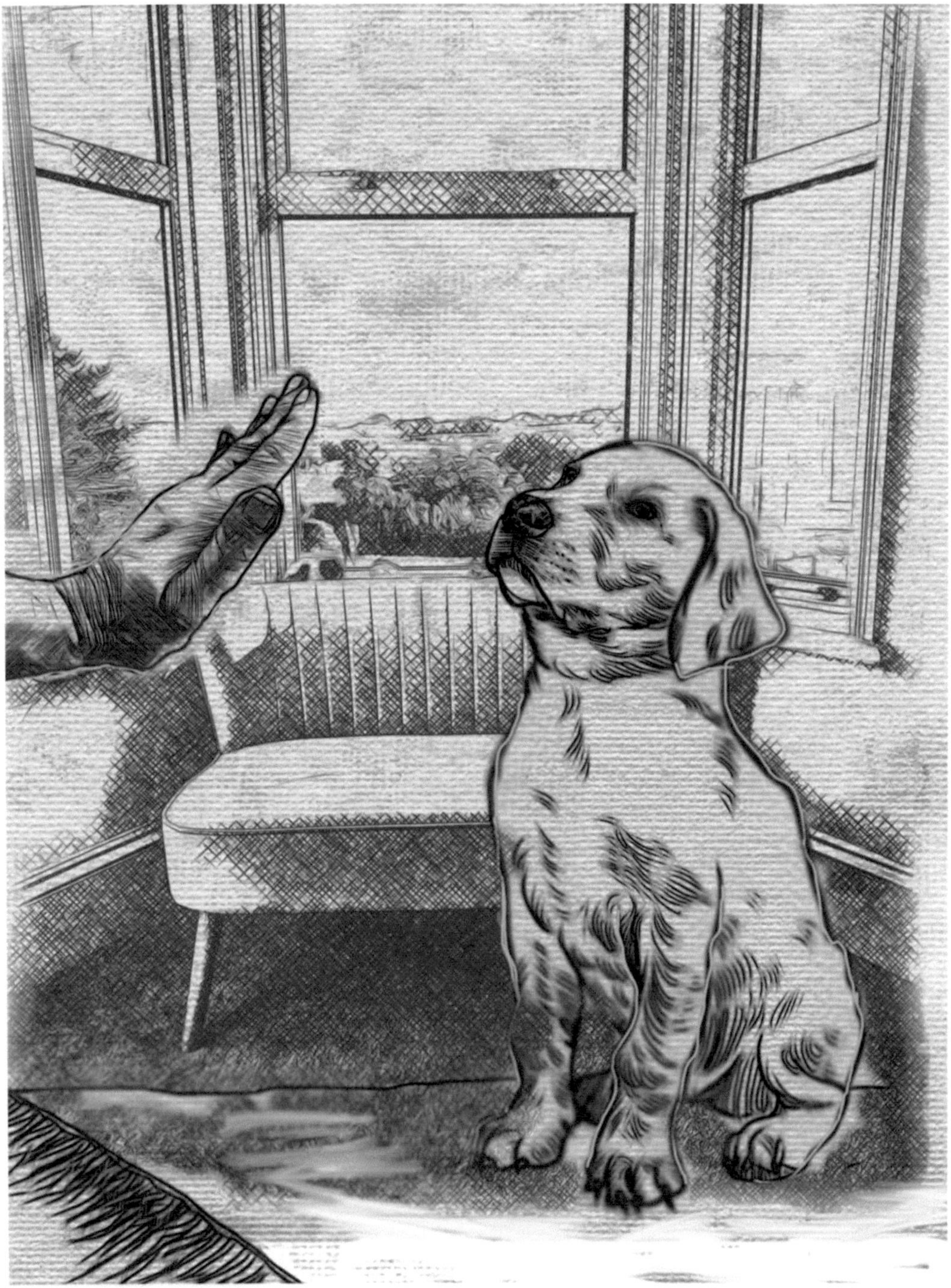

"Boundaries mean making it clear what is acceptable or unacceptable behaviour."

Chapter 10

Training: Your rules of the road

I imagine you're wondering what's the difference between boundaries and training? Well, there's an overlap certainly. As you've just read, boundaries revolve more around your doggie etiquette and what's deemed acceptable or unacceptable behaviour between you and your human.

Training is a bit more of a doggy boot camp affair (though I hope you won't be wearing any sort of footwear). Your human will teach you, sometimes with help from a professional, how to behave when you're out and about, both on and off the lead.

You will learn how to walk by your human's side, not 100 yards in front; you shouldn't pull them along, or dictate the pace. I know you youngsters find it very hard to refrain from pulling in your eagerness to explore all those exciting new smells and places, but refrain you must.

It's many moons ago, but I do remember the sheer excitement of going for a walk with my human. Let's be honest, it's probably one of the highlights of your day. It's natural to want to get going as quickly as possible, sniffing here, weeing there, zig-zagging to ensure nothing is missed. It really is a sensational sensory experience.

But that said, it's bad manners to be tugging and jumping about like a pooch on a pogo stick. Your human will need to curb your canine instinct to hit the ground running and tugging, paws akimbo. This is what training is all about.

You will be shown how to sit calmly while you have your lead or harness put on and off. You will be shown how to sit and wait with your human before crossing a road and to lie down if requested.

Now the bane of many of your humans' lives, is your recall. That means coming back to your human when they call you. This can take time, patience and persistence on your human's part. For you it's likely to involve some rather tasty treats and lots of praise when you do get it right. Some of you find this much easier to master than others.

Unfortunately, if your human hasn't the time or is a bit on the lazy side and doesn't put in the effort to help you with this, you'll be in for some serious canine confusion and delayed doggy dilemmas further down the line.

Without training you have no rules to follow

This is something many humans just don't get. It would be like 11 players running eagerly on to a pitch for an important football match, but there being no referee and no rules. Everyone is running for the ball, shouting and waving their arms, but no one knows which goal is theirs, which way they're supposed to be running, or even which players are on their side.

What a complete pickle and one destined to end in tears. If you don't receive appropriate training as a pup, you and your human will find yourselves in a similar predicament.

Without training you have no rules to follow. You're playing that football game at your own pace and probably at full throttle with your human being pulled along in your wake. Your human should assume the role of match referee. Their job is to ensure you follow the rules (that they've already explained to you during many hours of repetitive training).

If they do not, they're likely to be flailing around trying to control you, with elongated arms, strained backs and hoarse voices, in the process. They will become a very stressed person at the end of your lead. (In my humble canine view, even with a referee, rules, tactics and training, some football teams still appear not to have a clue when to run, kick or shoot, but I digress.)

Now unfortunately, as mad as it sounds, many humans don't actually get around to training you. I know, it sounds ludicrous and a very basic mistake to make, but make it they do, and in their thousands too. (I did warn you they tend to lack common sense.)

It's another anomaly that the British are renowned as a nation of dog-lovers. Their care and compassion for us canines far outweigh that of those from many other countries. But that care sometimes doesn't extend to making the effort to train you. This is another canine conundrum I find most baffling. For to me, it's part and parcel of humans doing their best for you.

Without training your human may find walking you quite challenging, especially if you're a strong specimen. You'll be eager to sniff left and right, forward and back. You'll want to run up to the nice-looking dog over there, or bark at the one who's not so nice over here. You'll be very eager to get going, rarely walking to heel, sitting or waiting.

You'll be charging through gates ahead of your human and generally being what your human might call a bloody nuisance, although no skin has been cut. You'll find the outside world full of wonders and scents that stimulate and excite you. That's why it's so vital your human trains you to gain some control for your own safety and that of other humans, dogs and animals.

Case study: Billy the Bullmastiff

Billy is a strong dog who wasn't trained to walk nicely on a lead. He tells Dr Peter Pointer how his human dad ended up in hospital when Billy's protective instincts took over.

"Dad was the only person who took me out for walks. The rest of the family said I was too strong and didn't do as I was told. I am bigger than most dogs. The vet says I weigh 59 kilograms. One evening when Dad and I were out in the dark, I saw a couple of men coming towards us. They were shouting and seemed to be fighting with each other. I didn't like the atmosphere around them and I felt Dad tense up on the end of my lead. Dad needn't have worried; I was quite ready to step in and protect him. As we drew closer, the men began shouting at Dad. That was enough for me. No one shouts at my dad in a nasty manner. I felt my hackles go up and I lunged forward barking. I was warning them off. It did the trick and they ran away. Unfortunately, I'd caught Dad unawares. He lost his balance and fell awkwardly. I didn't realise it at the time as I was in 'Defend Dad mode,' but I dragged him along as I chased the men. Dad was on the pavement, screaming in agony. His leg was at a funny angle and he couldn't move it. Apparently, it was broken and he had to go to hospital. After that Mum arranged for a professional dog trainer to teach me how to walk without pulling."

You are not stupid, you're untrained

Without training you may get labelled a difficult dog, an over-exuberant dog, or even a stupid dog. Now I'll tell you for nothing, you are not stupid, but you are untrained. You have no rules to follow, so have no choice but to do your own thing.

If blame is to be bandied about, there is only one door at which to lay it - the door of the human. They brought up said untrained and unruly dog through its puppy years, so with them the buck stops.

If your human hasn't shown you repeatedly, the behaviour they require of you when you're out on lead walks and when running free, how are you supposed to know?

You are very intelligent, but your natural instincts are to explore, often at top speed. If you're not taught any differently, or instilled with good manners, you'll behave as nature intended. That will be deemed at best, impolite and at worst, downright doggy delinquent.

If you're a pup arriving in your new home, it's likely your human will begin simple learnings with you straightaway. It's a good time for you to take it in as you're at your peak puppy learning stage at between 7 and 16 weeks. You'll soak up rules and regulations like a canine sponge. However, this critical learning period, coincides with your peak cutie puppy stage. This means it's the most high-risk time for your human to give in to your every whiny whim and, if you look at them adoringly enough, you may get away with almost anything.

You'll find your early learning always begins with what humans call house-training. This means ensuring you learn to go to the toilet outside, not on their best fluffy rug, cosy lounge carpet, or woe-betide you, on their bed.

You'll learn through cold, wet and windy experience, that your poos and wees must be done outside, even if it is raining or blowing a gale out there. You may not be used to this if your early weeks were spent in an outside building, or if your human breeder didn't begin the process.

If that's the case, you will find it very unsettling to be scooped up and dumped outside every hour or so. Even with the brightest of you and the best will in the world, you will have accidents. If you're in the arms of an experienced dog-owning human, they will take these wet and squidgy accidents in their stride - though hopefully executing a nifty, neat side-step over said accident. They won't make a big fuss and will make a note to self to be more watchful of you next time. They'll ensure they put you outside regularly and in good time so you can do your business, on the grass or patio or wherever is deemed your toileting area.

To help you to get to grips with this, your human will ensure you have access to the great (or small) outdoors at regular intervals. In these early days, you'll need to be watched like a hawk. You'll find you're desperate to wee after you've just woken up, after playing and after meals. If your human isn't paying attention, they will reap the wee-puddled, poo-piled consequences.

If they think about it properly, your toileting needs are very similar to theirs. You'll find they have a wee first thing in the morning and last thing at night. They'll also go several times during the day and after a big drink or meal. If they apply the same principles to you, as they would to a very young child, all will be well. If they leave you to your own devices, then I guarantee they will be stepping in puddles and sniffing out soft mounds of the brown stuff, with only their half-witted, careless selves to blame.

As an excited pup, eager to discover the world, you could be forgiven for thinking that this talk of training involves some sort of doggy duty in the canine army corps, but rest assured it's not. Now I'm sure that at three-months-old, you'll have many places to romp on your puppy bucket list. But, along with boundaries, it's vital your human puts in the training time.

If untrained you're like a car with no driver

Please forgive another vehicle analogy, but if a human started up a car, let out the clutch and pressed on the accelerator but hadn't learnt to drive, that's similar to having you as an untrained dog – of whatever age. With a good human at your side (in fact you should be at their side) who has taught you properly, you should both be well-equipped to face the big, wide, doggy and human world.

Training is also an opportunity for your human to get to know you better and to bond with you over a job well done. Your human will discover how rewarding it is to see you running full pelt towards them, ears akimbo, tongue a-lolling and tail aloft as you respond eagerly to their call, or whistle. They will feel real accomplishment (as will you), and you can revel in their praise when you get this right.

Depending on your breed, you'll probably take a few lessons and repetition to get to grips with things. But, in the right hands, it's very impressive what you can achieve. Note I say in the right hands. It will help you if your human learns what clear dog communication is.

If you're with an impatient human who bellows at you if you don't get it right, it will be much harder for you to learn. You'll end up feeling confused and possibly a little scared. Don't worry, that's not your fault.

Shouting and stomping never helped any pup learn anything. If your human is a novice to training, hopefully they will seek out a professional for help and advice. There are training classes and one-to-one lessons especially for puppies and rescue dogs, so with a bit of extra Lassie luck, your human will get you and them, booked into one of those.

An equally important part of your early training, is for you to get used to being left alone. Some humans fear you will die of heartache if they are not there to fuss around you. The truth is, if you're accustomed to quiet time from being a pup, you will be more than happy to be left alone.

You may find the humans who won't or don't coach you in this respect may fall into several categories.

a) They enjoy the fact that you crave their attention and need them
b) They lack the resolve to take the lead in your relationship
c) We're back to the old favourite, a lack of common sense.

Time-out from humans is good for you

Not only is it good for your mental well-being to have time out from hurly-burly human life, but you also need to learn that life doesn't always revolve around you. There are occasions when you need to be a good girl or boy and 'look after the house' while your human goes off to do non-dog-focused things.

Having a few hours quietly snoozing with no human interruptions, is actually quite a blessing. You can snuggle up in comfort, perhaps on the sofa or bed (if house rules allow), with bags of stretching, wriggling and rolling room and you won't be disturbed. You can fart to your heart (and bottom's) content, with no humans making loud laments of revolt, waving their hands back and forth and wrinkling up their noses.

You can sniff around the kitchen for fallen food without being shooed away; slurp your water as noisily as you like and splash it around as much as you please. You can generally 'dog out' without any human intervention. You should consider these home alone periods as valuable, human-free breaks in which to relax, unwind and recharge your doggy batteries. Living with humans can be a tiring affair, so welcome the opportunities for some 'you time' with open paws.

In the course of my studies, I've met many of you who have never been left alone by your human. I find this quite staggering – and I'm a pretty sure-pawed spaniel. If you're not acclimatised to being left as a puppy, it's likely to become a HUGE doggy deal as you get older. If the day comes when your human has to leave you, no doubt you'll feel very anxious. You may bark, whine, scratch at doors, chew furniture, or rip up carpets in an attempt to find your human and express your frightened feelings. You don't know if your human is coming back and you can't understand why, as the centre of their world, you're suddenly without them.

Humans call it separation anxiety and it is a condition that has become depressingly widespread. If you are into your twos or older and you've never kept house, it's quite likely your human will need professional help. Advice from a trainer or behaviourist will probably be required to avoid you getting yourself into a terrible lonesome tizzy.

Now I believe keeping house is a very important role and the more self-respecting among you, should be honoured to take it on. You are basically, the sole guardian of the human home. The human's property is being left completely in your protective, capable paws. Even if those paws have a heavy, sleepy head resting upon them, should an unwelcome visitor appear, you can bet your comfy bed you'll be up and at 'em before they can say "there's a good dog."

Over-socialisation can make you anxious

You may develop separation anxiety, if you're living with a human who has the unnecessary need to take you absolutely everywhere with them. (I call that over-socialisation.) Of course, you will happily trot along with them because that's what you do. But, if you have a nervous disposition, it can sometimes be an unsettling or downright uncomfortable experience.

For instance, if you're fearful of meeting other dogs, why take you to a dog show? That's your worst nightmare. If you are insecure among unknown humans, why take you to a busy shopping area or market?

Some humans believe you just have to get used to it. (Note that word 'just' again.) By making you face your fears, these humans hope, or expect you to get through it on your own. I'm sorry to say, they really don't understand your delicate doggie minds. In truth, all that will happen is your stress levels will likely go through the roof and you'll be even more nervous on your next outing.

The trouble is, you don't have any choice. Once you're in your harness, or on the end of a lead, you'll follow your human to the end of the earth if that's what they ask – but it doesn't mean you're enjoying the experience. Your human need only glance at your darting eyes, panting mouth, cowed demeanour and tightly tucked-in tail, to see you're a very unhappy dog in whatever uneasy situation you may find yourself in. This is when your human should respect your boundaries. Pushing you over lines that your paws would prefer not to cross is far from ideal.

Alas, the chances are, they're so busy buying something, chatting to friends, having a drink or generally enjoying themselves, they don't realise that you're not.

Case study: Georgie the German Shepherd

Georgie was bought by her dad as a pup during the human Covid-19 pandemic. They spent all their time together. She tells Dr Peter Pointer how she can't bear being left alone.

"I love my dad to bits. We do everything together and I'm always at his side. When he got me as a pup, the human world was closed so we spent all our waking and sleeping hours together in his house. Even when he was working at his laptop, I curled up by his feet. I rarely let him out of my sight. If ever he went out, he always took me with him. Sometimes he left me in the car, but that was ok because I knew he would be coming back. One day Dad told me he had to go into the office and I'd have to look after the house. I didn't really know what he meant, but I sensed something unusual was happening. He got his coat and car keys and I bounced about, ready to go too. But he didn't take me. As soon as he shut the front

door, I started to feel anxious. I began scratching at the door and whining. When he didn't come back, my anxiety turned to fear and then to panic. I began barking and wasn't really aware exactly what I was doing. I was just driven by this frantic desire to get through the door to find Dad. I ripped up the carpet, chewed apart some of the skirting board and shredded the door mat. I then tugged all the coats down off their hooks and began ripping them up. After what seemed like an age, I heard Dad's footsteps outside and his key in the lock. He had trouble opening the door because of all the mess I'd made. I was so pleased to see him I nearly knocked him over. He could see how frantic I'd been while he was out, but he didn't tell me off despite the damage. A few days later a nice lady came to the house. She was a dog behaviourist, whatever that is. I heard her telling Dad I'd spent too much time with him as a pup and not been taught to stand on my own four paws. She's going to show Dad how to help me with that. But first, Dad has to repair the front door, the coat hook, the skirting board and buy a new mat and carpet."

At your waggy doggie core, what drives most of you is an inherent desire to please your human. That's another huge difference between you and your human. Your love for them is utterly unconditional and your loyalty knows no bounds. (See Chapter 13 for more on love.)

If your human trains you in a clear and consistent manner your tail will wag for England, or whichever country you may find yourself in. The location is irrelevant, but there is no feeling like the one of utter pride and pleasure when you sit, lie, wait, heel, or fetch, as and when your human asks. Your human will feel pretty elated too, for it proves their training of you is paying off.

You'll also find that by working together in this way, the two of you build a strong connection. The more you train together, the stronger your bond develops with your human, becoming deep and long-lasting. You will want to do your best for them and they for you. It works both ways, that's the beauty of it.

There is a canine caveat here. The training you need is what humans call positive reinforcement - basically the praise and treats mentioned above. If you hear your human mention that phrase, you're on the right road. There are other training methods meted out by some humans (usually those bad beings), and I hope you never have to endure them. These involve using fear, force and physical aggression. I call them cruel.

I remember once meeting a gun dog who didn't lift its sad, brown eyes from the floor. With its head hung low and tail tucked in, it didn't take a Professor to know the way that poor dog had been trained. It was heart-breaking to see. It may have been doing everything it was told (it wouldn't dare do anything different), but it was a very unhappy dog. Its spirit had been broken by force and fear.

If your human likes to shout and wave their arms, usually in frustration, you'll get confused and panicky, unsure what they want you to do. A human who loses their temper with you and blames you into the bargain, shouldn't be attempting to train you. You'll learn best with a patient, calm and enthusiastic approach, so you too feel excited and eager to learn. If your human is of the short-tempered, shouty variety, the only thing

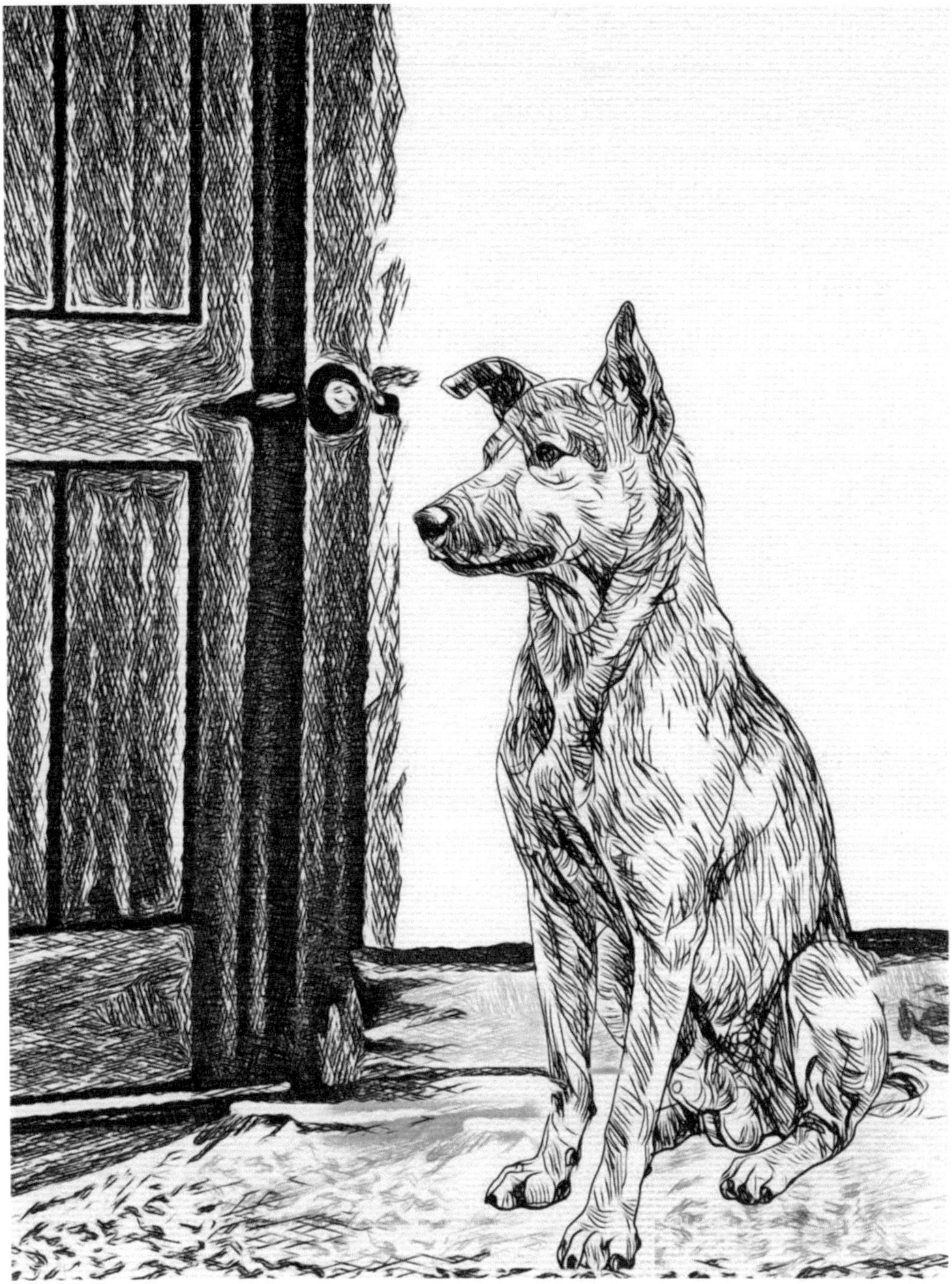

"Keeping house is a very important role and you should feel honoured to take it on."

they'll accomplish is overloading your doggy senses, making you fearful and unable to absorb new information.

I'm not going into the whys and wherefores of canine training, as that isn't my field – though fields are an important part of it. Dog training and behaviour has become a big issue here in the UK, with entire television series devoted to the matter. These programmes usually highlight some extremely badly behaved Bulldog or picky Pomeranian. It soon becomes evident that sadly, their human hasn't set any boundaries or done any effective training. The lives of this desperate human and demon dog have reached breaking point.

With the input of the expert, the confounded human learns some basic dos and don'ts and within days, the once uncontrollable canine has become the best-behaved, bow-wow on the street. The stressed human, previously at their nitwits end, is transformed into one of smiling serenity, sweetness and light – all thanks to some simple training and clear boundaries.

Professor Daniel's Bones of Retention:

- **Some humans won't train you**
- **Time alone to chill out is good for you**
- **Looking after the house is an honour**
- **You'll learn quicker when keen**
- **Being untrained is not your fault**
- **Avoid short-tempered, 'shouty' trainers**
- **Pleasing your human is a great feeling**

Chapter 11

Socialisation: Wagging your way into the world

Now here's a doggy dichotomy for you. In the previous chapter, I explained how it's extremely important that as a young dog you learn to look after the house on your own. So, prick up those ears because this next lesson is just as important, but the complete canine opposite – it's about learning to leave the house to go out and about.

Just when you think you've cracked the house-training and are happy snoozing in your cosy corner, you'll be flung into the frantic and often scary scenario of the ever-moving, ever-grooving, big wide human world. It's certainly quite a place, but it's one in which you need to feel as comfortable and ideally, as calm as possible. So be prepared to put your surest paws forward and don your strongest, Superdog pants.

If you thought living with a human was hard, prepare to have your hound-stinct well and truly tested. Humans calls this puppy socialisation. It's a big word, but it needs to play an equally large and important part in your early life.

Your first few months are the critical times for your human to be introducing you to all the exciting things the world has in sniffy store for you. Once you leave the comfort of your natural mum's warm and milky teat, you will discover for yourselves what a world of wonder awaits you.

From ear-splitting car horns and piercing house alarms, to wailing emergency sirens and the roar of trains and HGVs. Initially your human may appear surprised if you back off, shake and cower in the presence of these deafening and quite frankly, petrifying daily accompaniments to human lives.

Noisy street monsters can be pretty scary

Humans, of course, are immune to these monsters in the street and they may not appreciate that to you they seem pretty scary. Some may rebuke you for your silly actions. You may find yourself hauled along in your harness, or semi-choked as you're tugged lead-first past them.

If they were to put themselves in your paws for a moment, they would see that you need their understanding, support and encouragement when you experience these scenarios for the first-time.

If you're of a sensitive doggy disposition, you may freeze on the spot, or try to wriggle away in a speedy snake-like fashion. In this case, your human may need to take things more slowly. (Whether they do or don't, is a bit of a goofy gamble, but forcing you into a scary space is never a good idea.)

If you're of a more confident nature, you may be completely unfazed. As long as your human is at your side and says it's ok, then as far as you're concerned, it is.

As you venture wider into the human world, you'll hear, see and smell all sorts of things you could never have imagined. Humans eat some very scent-laden food - they often leave it lying around too. You'll likely sniff out discarded chips and half-eaten pasties. (Professional Daniel's tip: Avoid the curry sauce.) Your human will need to keep their wily wits about them to protect you from the perils of this dubious pavement food.

Talking of food, if your locality has a pet shop, that's usually excellent news and worth barking about. It means you could well be in for some regular treats. Pet shops are packed with all-things animal, largely doggy. They are often run by generous animal-lovers, so you will be made very welcome. If you go in to say hello, you'll probably receive a treat or a biscuit, as there's often a large jar on the counter.

They'll hope that once inside, your unsuspecting human will indulge you, buying some special snacks. While your human chats and chooses, you can search the shelves as you munch happily on your biscuit, sniffing out the latest offers.

You'll meet creatures great and small

If you live in a rural area there will be a colourful crowd of unusual and large creatures, both farmed and wild, who you'll need to meet, calmly and quietly in a controlled manner. Ideally your meet and greet will be done with you on a lead or harness and behind a fence. You're likely to come nose-to-nose with big-eyed, moo-ing cows, long-legged horses with clattering hooves and foot-stomping ewes protecting their lambs.

You may even find yourself face-to-face with those long-necked and camel-like creatures that hail from the hills of Peru in South America. They're known as llamas and alpacas and are kept by some farmers. They look very strange creatures to me, a cross between a sheep and a camel. Word on the field is they can be a bit flighty and sensitive. Beware the longer-legged llama as they are not averse to meting out a well-aimed kick if they're scared or upset. They also have a dirty habit of spitting.

Many of you will be eager to chase the scampering rabbits and squirrels, or see off the squawking pheasants and screeching, swooping birds that you'll discover down those country lanes and fields. Humans call these creatures wildlife and whether you're allowed to indulge in an exciting game of chase, will very much depend on your mum or dad.

Case study: Harry the Huntaway

Harry hadn't been introduced to many animals when he was young. He tells Dr Peter Pointer how his excitement at meeting a mystery creature nearly cost him his life.

"I was having a lovely walk with Mum and Dad out in the country. We lived in a town so it was great to be away from the roads and traffic. I was off-lead running about, when I saw this big animal up ahead. It was standing behind a wooden fence. It had very long, slim legs and a long nose. Its ears were short and pointy and it had tousled hair down its neck and a swishy tail. I didn't know what it was, but wondered if it would like to play. I ran towards it, eager to say hello. As I approached, it looked down at me, snorted and threw up its head. I took that as a good sign, so squeezed through the fence, wagging my tail. I could hear Mum and Dad calling my name, but I was busy with my new friend. I bowed down to it and barked and suddenly the animal took off, kicking its back legs up in the air. I thought this looked like a great game, so I began to play chase. I was amazed at how quick it moved, but I managed to keep up. Then it stopped, as suddenly as it had started and began rearing up on its back legs. I looked up

and noticed its feet had hard-looking shoes on. The rearing up took me by surprise as its front legs came thundering down right by me. I darted to one side but then it turned and began kicking out at me with its back legs. I felt a gush of wind whistle past my head as this animal's foot missed me by a whisker. Then I caught Mum's voice screaming my name in a tone of real fear and desperation. In that instant I realised this animal wasn't playing chase and didn't actually want me there at all. It was trying to hurt me. So I turned tail and shot back out under the fence, the animal thundering after me. Mum was crying and Dad was both pleased and cross with me. I heard them saying, "but he's never seen a horse before." So that's what it was. Since then, I've given horses a very wide berth."

Be wary of claw-wielding cats

One domestic beast of which you should be particularly wary is the unpredictable, claw-wielding cat. If you find yourself in a household that's already home to a feline or two, I'd advise you to steer well clear.

They can be all sweetness and purring light one minute, then boxing you around the face with their needle-like sharp claws the next. Some are downright snooty and will simply ignore you. Others are of the spitty and hissy variety. I've met several unsuspecting canines who have been on the receiving end of an attack from one of these. You don't even have to put a paw wrong to upset them. Felines find it fun to torment and tease innocent young dogs. I think they realise you are still learning the laws of the animal land, so they like to lord their experience over you. At best, you may sustain a sharp scratch;

at worst, you may suffer a damaged cornea or scarred, bleeding nose. Be warned.

If you're a very small dog, meeting larger breeds in a calm manner will help give you confidence. Introducing you to a gentle giant of a sociable dog in a controlled and organised way will show you big doesn't mean bad. It will help you accept larger dogs without fear or recoil. In time you may find they become some of your best doggy friends.

Whether you are a bear-like St Bernard or a Miniature Dachshund, the same doggie boundaries and training apply. Size of paws and girths of snouts are irrelevant, for you all carry the same canine instinct inside you.

As your human widens your view of the world, you'll discover rivers are great for sploshing, salty seas for swimming, deep lakes for doggy-paddling, and muddy ponds and puddles to plonk down in belly-first.

Prepare also, to find your paws padding across all sorts of strange surfaces. Unfortunately, the human world isn't made up of our much-preferred cooling green grass and dusty dirt tracks. Out there, you will find unforgiving concrete and tarmac that's hard enough to scratch the pads off a panther, let alone an enthusiastic young dog.

You'll come across what humans call bridges. Strange and unusual structures that stretch across rivers and roads. Being at a height with moving objects below you, can be quite an unnerving experience - whatever your age. I must admit, I'm not a fan myself, never have been. So, it's another time when you'll need to take a deep breath, put your best paws forward and be guided by, and stick like glue to your trusty human.

You'll be warmly welcomed in many places

Today, you'll find many venues frequented by your humans will warmly welcome you too. (I'm thinking cafes, restaurants, pubs and retail outlets.) As with pet shops, there will be tasty doggy treats and shiny drinking bowls available, especially for you. I've even heard of dedicated doggie menus in some establishments. Once upon a time, when I was a pup, such notions weren't entertained. Either I was left in a chilly kennel in the backyard, or tied up outside said shop or pub until my human's purchasing, or drinking and eating business was done.

When it comes to socialising, you may discover your human will use *you* to help *them* meet other people. With a dog at their side, humans who lack confidence, or feel a little uncomfortable in social settings, often feel better by simply having you at their side. Think of yourself as their four-legged, moral support. Never underestimate how important that can be to a human. With you as the focus, rather than them, it takes the heat off your clammy-handed human. They can relax while you happily take centre stage, canine-style, in any human interactions.

You'll also notice that rather than greeting each other with a sensible bottom-sniff, humans make small-talk. This is usually nonsense chit-chat about the weather, their health or where they live. (If they were more like us, they could learn all this with a simple whiff of the other's back end in a few seconds.)

However, with you at their side, the chances are you will feature highly in the conversation. They will discuss your age, breed, how long you've been with your human, any background or rescue history, and hopefully, what a good dog you are. If the other human also has a dog and the two of you get on, the opportunities are endless for new friendships to be forged and partnerships to grow.

In fact, some humans enjoy socialising together so much, they may forget you're even there. Many a time I've seen humans happily walking and talking, so utterly engrossed, they've no idea what you and the rest of the pack are up to. You may be relieving yourself of last night's dinner, getting into a tussle with a less sociable dog on its lead, or rolling vigorously in some pungent poo. Your happy humans, coffee cups in hands, stride ahead oblivious. Meanwhile, your poo is left steaming on the footpath, the owner of the unsociable dog is left tangled and distraught, and the formerly clean and once yellow poo-roller is now a new shade of stinky black.

Today, the world is very welcoming of humans with dogs, but it's not always possible for you to go everywhere. Let's face it, would you really want to attend a black-tie dinner? (Though admittedly there would be rich pickings under the tables.) A college prize-giving with much loud clapping and no food in sight is no fun for you. Similarly, a noise-pumping, strobe-dazzling music festival is the last place for your sensitive eyes and ears.

As well as shopping trips, evenings out and other dog-free events, you'll find there will be longer periods of time when your human has to leave you and their home. This is another good reason to learn to be your own dog and stand firmly on your own four paws.

Humans may take you on holiday

Whereas you and I see every day as one to be enjoyed to the maximum with walks, games, food, cuddles and fun, humans have designated weeks in the year when they focus on doing this. They call these periods holidays and they usually last a week or two, sometimes more.

It's a time when your human seeks out warmer, sunnier, or even wetter, colder places to live. Some humans take their holidays in the UK, some go by car or plane to hotter places abroad. Depending which your human chooses, you could find yourself bundled into the boot, passport in paw to join them.

If not, you could be taking a different type of holiday in a dog hotel or boarding house. Often described as a home from home, they are basically another dog-lover's house. There, you'll be able to lounge around in chairs or on sofas, stretch out on a rug in front of a fire and meet other sociable dogs on their holidays.

Other options could see you spending your holiday at a relative's house, having a friend or paid dog-sitter moving in to the comfort of your own home, or being cared for at a kennels.

Even for the most balanced of dogs, this holiday period can be a little unsettling, especially for the first few times. There's always the concern of whether your human will return to you or not. Again, if you're introduced to this holiday scenario as a pup, you are more likely to trot off happily on your solo sojourn.

If you have been trained and socialised, you'll be happy mixing with new friends on your doggy holiday. Meeting charming new canines is always fun and hours of happy holiday rompings and outdoor fun and games await.

In the run-up to this holiday, you may notice your humans getting very stressed. Suitcases will appear from under beds, or out of attics and summery clothes and toiletries will be piled high on the side. This is your human frantically preparing to go on holiday.

At this stage, you will no doubt get under their feet, as you'll be picking up on their stress and worrying what is going on. Trotting around anxiously behind them won't be popular. In fact, they're likely to take their stress out on you when they've misplaced their new bikini, or fruitlessly hunted high and low for their favourite flip-flops. (Whatever you do, leave this strange rubbery, flippy floppy footware alone. Though I admit, it's exceedingly chewable, I can guarantee that unlike the soft-soled summer foot attire, you won't be flavour of the month.)

On your human's return, there will be a similarly frantic few days when they are catching up with washing, opening post and preparing for the return to work, school and social life. Despite your eagerness to be reassured, your best bet is to lie low during these pre and post-holiday preparations and wait for life to return to normal, whatever that means for you. However, when sharing your life with humans, my experience is there is no such thing as normal.

Children can be unpredictable and unkind

When being socialised, you're likely to come across little humans called children. Now a gentle word of warning here. They can be unpredictable and sometimes unkind. If you're living with a best buddy type of human, they will have the common sense to know children, especially young ones, should never be left alone with you. An adult human – and ideally one with half a brain – should always be keeping a watchful eye if you and young children are together. I would say it's not so much because of what you might do, but more the child.

The trouble with young children, is they're likely to run at you full force, whether you want them to or not. They may pull your ears, poke you in the eye, tug your tail, stand on your paws, or even try to ride you like a horse. Some will dress you up in human clothes and, whether you are prepared to allow any or all of this, will depend very much on your upbringing, your temperament, your life history and your breed.

If you are a rescue dog who was physically abused in a former home, you will probably not take too kindly to being pummelled and pulled about by some unsupervised child. (And who can blame you. It may trigger unpleasant memories you don't wish to revisit.)

If you've always lived in a quiet home with an elderly human, you will be understandably wary of noisy, energetic little humans. Their high-pitched screams and squeals are likely to set your molars on edge. Their sudden and quick movements are far removed from the sedate shufflings you're used to. You'll probably feel a little anxious, fearful even, unsure what these uncontrolled, imp-like beings may do next. You can't read them and don't understand what's going on.

If you're unhappy with a child's behaviour and you are able to withdraw quietly from such unstable surroundings, I'd advise you to do so as soon as you can. If your human is nearby, go and hide behind them and they may realise your reluctance to want to play with these squeaky little people.

If you're feeling cornered or threatened, you may give warnings that you're unhappy with the situation. You'll feel your head tense up, your ears go down, and it's likely that the whites of your eyes will appear (though you, of course, won't see this yourself). If you're feeling very unsure, and you are unable to retreat, you may feel obliged to growl and curl up your lip. Don't feel you are the monster here. This change in your behaviour is simply you showing the usual canine warning signs of perceived threat and danger.

Humans need to heed your warnings

The risk comes if humans do not notice and heed your warnings. Children are too young to read you (even some adult humans can't). It is the responsibility of the adult human in the home to put an end to the scary scenario in which you find yourself. They need to remove either you, or the child, from the situation.

If you are unable to move somewhere that feels safe for you, things can quickly escalate. If no intervening action is taken and the threat towards you heightens, your last resort will be to snap or snarl, possibly even bite or attack, and no one wants that.

Case study: Romeo the Romanian crossbreed

Romeo was a Romanian street dog who was brought to the UK by a charity. He was rehomed by a couple who'd not had a dog before. He told Dr Peter Pointer how, most of the time, he lives in fear.

"I've not lived in a house before and I've not had much contact with humans either, so both these things frighten me. Luckily my humans have some outdoor space so I stay out there as much as possible. I'm scared of them touching me and I hate being shut in the house at night. The charity staff got me used to wearing a harness, but I find going out with my humans very overwhelming. My ears are always flat and I drop my head in the hope no one will notice me. My humans regularly take me out when I'd rather stay quietly in the garden. I hear them telling other humans I'm from Romania. They take me to shops and pubs which I find noisy and claustrophobic. It makes me feel really anxious. I don't like being on the lead and I don't like being indoors with lots of humans. One day we were in a cafe. It was very small and I had to sit under a table. I saw all these human legs coming and going and there was lots of clattering and banging. I felt really panicky. My humans didn't seem to notice, but I was panting with nerves and felt quite shaky. Then from nowhere, this little human came running towards me, squealing. I had nowhere to go as I was trapped under the table against a wall. I could feel my lips curling up and I heard a nasty growl come out of my mouth as I bared my teeth. Before my terror really took hold of me, the little girl's mum pulled her away from me. My humans were quite shocked that I'd reacted like that and told me off. I don't think they appreciate how very scared I am being in all these small, busy places with humans. If only they gave me more time and space."

Today, there are far too many tragic outcomes when dogs of dubious background are mixed with unsupervised little humans. Adult humans too, are not immune from feeling the fangs of a frightened canine in volatile, high-risk circumstances. I will stick my Spaniel neck out here and say, in my view, dog and human altercations are nearly always due to some degree of inappropriate human behaviour somewhere along the doggy line.

There may have been a deficit in your training, or an absence of boundaries. You may have been encouraged to behave over-protectively, or even aggressively by your human, probably a bad being type. All, or one of these issues can result in such sorry incidents of human injury and sometimes fatality from uncontrolled, dog behaviour. No dog wants to intentionally hurt a human for no good reason, especially those of you who live cosy, domesticated lives.

Some of you do have more protective traits, or are more sensitive to your surroundings, depending on your breed. Others of you will be in sheer bliss, snuggling up to a child on the sofa, or playing chase with teenagers in the garden. If your human does their research, they will know which of you are, or aren't best-suited to live with a family.

Above all, to feel comfortable and happy in a family environment, you need to be well-socialised as a pup, taught clear boundaries and repeated training, so you know what behaviour is and isn't acceptable to your human.

Professor Daniel's Bones of Retention:

- **Four sure paws are a great asset**
- **Keep your Superdog pants at the ready**
- **The human world is loud and scary**
- **Pet shops are full of free biscuits**
- **Beware hissy, spitty felines**
- **Children can be unpredictable**
- **Growling does not make you a 'monster'**

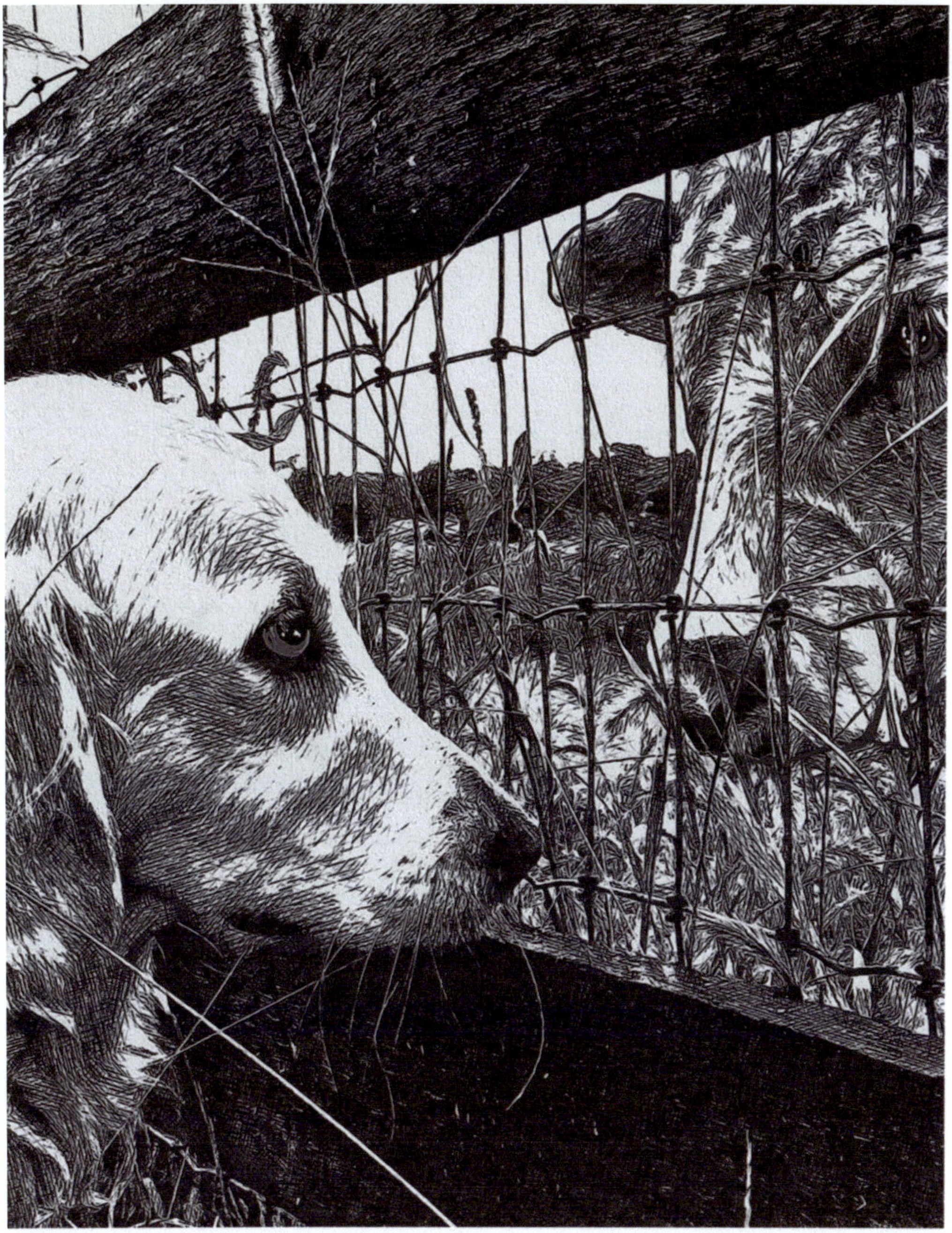

"Venturing into the human world, you'll hear, see, smell and meet all sorts of things – and creatures."

Chapter 12

Your Houndy Happiness: A healthy mind and body

One of the single, greatest influences on your mental health, or to put it simply, your ultimate, houndy happiness, is the human who shares your life.

Your breed will have a bearing on your propensity to feel fearful, or protective, crave physical exercise, or mental stimulation. You can't do much about this. It's in your DNA and that's just who you are. It's down to your human to ensure that whatever breed you are, they can fully meet your barkingly-detailed brief, for both your welfare and theirs.

Whether you feel anxious or safe, bored or fulfilled, ignored or included, fighting fit or in poor health, can be affected by the choices your human makes on your behalf. More often than not, these choices are out of your paws. The best you can do, is make your feelings known loudly and clearly by your behaviour. But of course, there's no guarantee your human will notice, understand, or act on it.

These choices cover everything from your exercise regime and training, to the collar or harness you wear, the food you're fed, your home environment and your physical health. Your well-being is affected, among other things, by any drugs you're given, the quality of your food and the type and frequency of treats.

Those of you who are strong and energetic and aren't trained to walk nicely to heel, risk damaging your necks if you wear a collar and lead. If you're constantly pulling and jerking on your cervical spine, you may harm it. You could bruise your muscles and adversely affect the major nerves in the neck, or even your thyroid. You may even restrict blood and energy flow between your head and neck, creating all manner of abnormal symptoms affecting everything from your eyes and ears to your limbs and skin.

Being yanked by your neck is no fun at all

I see many of you, pulling your humans along like some possessed, snow-bound, sled-dog. You're coughing and choking away like an old human with a cigarette addiction. At the very least, you're likely to return home with a hoarse throat and sore neck. (By hoarse I mean croaky, not the throat of a creature that goes clippety-clop.)

Being yanked about by the neck, is no fun at all. If your human puts their hands tightly around their own neck, then pulls it forcibly and suddenly, this way and that, they'll feel for themselves the discomfort and potential pain it can cause. It's not a pleasant predicament to be in.

Other physical damage can occur if, as a pup, your human over-exercises you. They risk damaging your delicate, undeveloped limbs. Some humans will be keen to take you out and about, thinking nothing of taking you on an arduous hill hike. They may even find it amusing to watch you plodding about with your floppy paws, trying to keep up. If you're allowed to clamber up and down stairs, on and off sofas and beds or if you have to scramble, cartoon-like, on smooth shiny floors with no grip, your human is putting your developing joints at risk of serious damage.

Dr Peter Pointer has this to say about vulnerable, growing limbs:

"The growth plates in the bones of puppies' legs, don't fuse until they are between 12 – 24 months-old, depending on the breed. This is why, as puppies, you plod about looking so sweet and clumsy. The growth plates are still open and your limbs extremely vulnerable to injury. If, as a puppy, you are over-exercised and damage a limb, you could end up deformed, or with an abnormal gait, for the rest of your life.

"Injury or damage may occur through high impact activity, such as long walks, ball or frisbee throwing and vigorous play. Damage at a young age, can also affect the growth and development of the rest of your bones and muscles. Over-exercising you as a puppy carries a very real health risk that needs to be taken seriously by your human."

Ball-throwing can make you obsessive

I explained earlier the risks to you if your human uses a ball-thrower. I make no apologies for reiterating that warning here. Aside from the potential physical injuries I mentioned, repeated ball-throwing can also affect your state of mind. By this I mean you're at risk of becoming obsessive and developing guarding behaviour. As you prance about, eager to chase and fetch, your adrenalin levels run high and so do your emotions. (We're back to that game of football. Think local Sunday league, usually featuring much shouting and gesticulating.) For you this translates as barking incessantly at your human to keep throwing said ball. More often than not they will oblige, thinking you're enjoying it, rather than obsessing over it.

For you that hurled ball is your prized possession. It has your complete focus. So how do you feel when some cocky Cavapoo fancies a slice of your chase and catch action? It's likely that you won't be impressed. How you show your displeasure can vary from a warning growl or snarl, to a snapping of teeth in their direction or, a full-on bite.

If ball-chasing is your daily exercise, your body has no chance to fully recover from these adrenalin rushes. You're likely to feel on alert all the time and unable to relax. In time you become an anxious dog who can't settle and needs professional help.

Another factor that can affect your mental and physical health is your diet. If you're fed kibble that's full of cereal, fillers and other unknowns you'll be unlikely to ever feel your tail-wagging best. Like humans, a poor diet can leave you lacking nutrients, or feeling hyper - and always hungry. You may have a dull, scurfy coat and loose, smelly poos. For some, your behaviour may be affected. You may be described as mad or over-exuberant, when in reality, you're eating a daily dose of over-processed pap.

Some treats do you more harm than good

The same goes for treats. I can put my paw on my heart and say that in my experience, the cheaper, or more attractive-looking they appear to humans, the fuller they are likely to be of artificial additives, colourings and other hu-manufactured nonsense.

Clever marketing makes some humans believe they're buying you a treat of exceptional value. In reality, your bargain chew, bone or other goodie could do you more harm than good. I've heard of dogs nearly choking on cheap rawhide chews, masquerading as treats.

Talking of treats, you may find your human is one of those generous souls who feeds you a steady stream of sausage slices or salmon sticks. Being so lovingly liberal with these delicious doggy delights is, on one paw, to be applauded. As we all know, it would be most rude to refuse a proffered titbit. But on the other paw, you're at risk of piling on the pounds and developing health-related issues associated with obesity.

If your human doesn't make mealtime adjustments – and by that, I mean giving you a little less breakfast, lunch or dinner – you're at risk of becoming one of those out-of-condition, podgy pooches. We've all seen them. Their belly swings low, their breathing is heavy and their poor joints are jarring under the weight of their porcine proportions. (I've also noticed that those of you who do end up in this porky predicament often live with humans who are themselves robust and rotund.) It's likely your human has an issue with boundaries around food, so may benefit from reading Chapter 9.

Personally, I like nothing better than some raw meat and a good bone now and again. When I changed my own diet from kibble to meat, I lost weight; my digestion and bowel movements improved and rarely do I have flatulence now – something a lot of your humans would really appreciate. I also have fewer bowel movements, producing only compact and dry waste. Another benefit when your human clears up after you.

I do understand that not all your humans are in a position to feed you a raw diet. As with so many canine-associated costs, they are ever-rising. I know some of you are in the very privileged position of having your meals prepared for you by hand, at home, but I don't think this is commonplace. I'm sure your human will do the best they can for you to suit their lifestyle and within their budget.

The human pandemic was a stressful time

Now, it's widely accepted that the global Covid-19 pandemic led to a surge in humans buying puppies, especially in the UK. They considered it a good time to take a pup into their homes. Humans were confined to barracks, could settle in, train, fuss and play with them.

However, I would proffer that if you were one of those pandemic pups, it was possibly the worst time to join a household. The family was out of its normal routine, and for some people the Covid period was itself a stressful experience. There were no opportunities for you to socialise or for your human to receive professional, one-to-one support, or attend group training classes.

For some humans, it was also the first-time they'd welcomed a dog into their home. This combination of unhelpful canine factors, meant some of you pandemic pups, have grown into rather anxious, unsocialised animals. You may find other dogs and the outside world rather scary.

Many humans became unnerved themselves during this strange pandemic period. Even if you were a well-established, 'old paw' in 2020, you could well have picked up on your human's stress.

Today, their society is one with many personal and financial pressures and some bizarre media and celebrity norms. Humans inhabit an image-conscious existence with a materialistic culture of which we canines, thankfully, have no understanding. But be aware, it puts huge mental pressure on some of them – and this could spill over on to you too.

If, for whatever reason, you are of an anxious disposition or from a traumatised background, there are many ways your human can support you. Taking advice from your vet is their best starting point. Enlisting the help of a canine behaviourist or trainer is another option.

Enabling you to do things that you enjoy, can help regulate your nervous system. I've already mentioned sniffing games and trails, flyball fun and agility, and for working breeds such as Labradors and Spaniels, there are gun dog activities – as long as you are working alongside a kind human with a heart.

Holistic help is available if you feel overwhelmed

There are also holistic therapies and solutions that can help, if you're a distressed doggy soul. Humans may not realise it, but they don't have the monopoly on natural remedies. If your human goes online, they'll find a range of herb-based supplements available for all manner of doggie ailments, mental and physical. Valerian and Skullcap, known for their calming properties on humans, are popular herbs in doggy supplements, for those of you feeling overwhelmed by the world. I believe they can be very effective to help calm an unsettled doggie mind. Your vet should be able to advise your human on this.

Now massage may be an unlikely therapy to spring to a human's mind, if seeking help for you during a stressful period. But, take it from me, it helps. I have known many an unhappy hound whose traumatised tremblings have been stilled by a course of sympathetic bodywork.

One specific type of massage that I'd like to mention, is called Whole Energy Body Balance (WEBB.) It's very effective at easing tension and silent pain, caused by both emotional and physical issues that you may have. It helps calm your quaking nerves, encouraging your body from its sympathetic nervous system (your fight or flight mode), into its parasympathetic nervous system (your rest and digest mode.) I've seen even anxious dogs stretched out in a deep relaxation by the end of a therapy.

Case study: Biddy the Border Terrier

Biddy was a happy girl until her human mum had to leave her to work abroad. Biddy went to live with a relative, but pined terribly. When her mum returned, six months later, Biddy was very anxious.

"I was absolutely delighted when Mum came home. I was so excited I did a little wee on the floor, which is something I never do. But I didn't feel quite right. Having Mum disappear from my life really unsettled me. I had no idea when or if she was coming back. I never really relaxed and spent a lot of time looking out of the window, hoping to see her. Mum noticed the change in me and

could see I wasn't the happy-go-lucky girl I'd been before she left. She told me not to worry, she was going to make me feel better. A few days later, we went to see a lady in a wooden cabin. Mum sat in a chair and I sat on a very comfortable, spongy bed. The lady sat on the floor and Mum told her all about me. The lady began stroking me very slowly. It felt nice, but I was a bit anxious. I was worried Mum might leave me again. I also wasn't sure what the lady was going to do, or if she might inject me, so I stayed on alert. Both Mum and the lady were very calm which helped me. The lady began gently feeling down my spine and putting pressure here and there. Some areas felt quite sore. I heard her tell Mum I was holding a lot of tension in different areas of my body. I didn't want to relax and let my guard down, but my physical body was beginning to melt under the massage. It felt very nice. After a while, I decided the lady wasn't going to inject me after all and actually seemed quite nice. I felt some bits of me flicking about as the lady massaged different parts of me. It was painful in places, but it also felt good to be free of the tightness. I felt my eyes going heavy and my head nodding. Mum encouraged me to lie down, which I did. I began to relax and let out a few deep sighs as the lady continued massaging me. I think I woke up about half an hour later. When I got home, I went straight to bed and slept like a log for the first time in six months. The next day I felt much lighter and happier. My back felt much freer too and I skipped about as I hadn't done for months. Mum took me back to the cabin lady for another two massages after that. She told the lady she had her 'happy girl' back and I've realised I don't feel anxious anymore."

Another holistic therapy that I rate highly is veterinary acupuncture. A specially-trained vet will gently insert very fine needles into meridians on your body. It may sound a little uncomfortable, but believe me it's very effective for a whole host of health issues.

Energy work is a further option if you've any past issues. It's an unlikely route for many humans who usually need to see things to believe them. For those open to such things, it can prove extremely enlightening for your human and very effective for you. But a word of warning - your human must find an experienced and registered energy worker. As with all walks of doggy and human life, some people are more skilled and effective than others.

Canine communicators can also help bring relief to those of you feeling misunderstood, mistreated and whose voices haven't been heard. These exceptionally advanced humans, can tune into your energy field, be it through seeing images, internal feelings, a clear knowing or even hearing. You can actually communicate with these humans and show or tell them what's in your heart and mind. This alone will help lighten your heavy emotional load.

Once you've unburdened yourself of whatever dark times you've been through, or whatever worries are weighing you down, you will feel lighter and happier in spirit and I bet my best beefy marrowbone that your human will begin to see positive changes in your behaviour and demeanour.

You're not just a dog

Being shown respect by your human and honouring you as the sensitive, intelligent creature that you are, can easily be overlooked in today's rather self-centred, human society. As I said previously, you are not 'just a dog' and any human who thinks such a thing, should never be allowed to share their home with you.

I'd love to see human legislators reintroduce licensing for those who wish to have you as companions. In my humble view, humans should have to attain a certain level of knowledge and understanding about your needs, before being allowed to take you into their home.

I know that some charities do excellent work educating children on how to care for and treat animals, especially dogs and cats. This is something I whole-heartedly applaud. Respecting and treating you as a dog (not a human, not a baby, a fur-baby, or a doll) is vital to your well-being. For instance, if you are sound asleep in your bed after a two-hour hill hike, you won't want to be hauled out to play like a favourite toy, by some demanding seven-year-old who wants a game of tug-of-war.

If you're tucking into your breakfast or dinner, you don't want it suddenly whipped away from you in some ill-judged joke. I've heard how some of you have been made to perform a 'hind leg dance' for minutes on end, putting unnecessary pressure on your hips in a bizarre begging ritual to qualify for a treat or toy. In the worst cases, you may be teased or taunted. In such a scenario, you're not actually given said treat or toy, despite your best begging efforts. You may be encouraged to carry out all sorts of undignified and unnatural canine paw-steps to earn your coveted prize.

Your half-witted human finds this unnatural doggie behaviour funny and entertaining. Of course, you do what they ask, because you want to please your human and more than anything, you also want that treat. But being encouraged (and doing) something unnatural for reward, doesn't mean you're enjoying it. In my view, it's demeaning and disrespectful. You're not a toy to be used for entertainment. Teasing you, or indeed any animal, is never acceptable.

If you're scared of water, throwing you into a pond, or squirting you with a hosepipe isn't amusing. It will serve only to heighten your watery fears.

If your country is experiencing high temperatures with scorching sunshine, a walk in the heat of the day is the last thing on your mind. Time and again I've seen humans, sweating it out in shorts and vests, dragging you along, insisting you go for a nice walk. Some of you will, understandably and quite rightly, try to retreat, sit down and do your utmost to resist. Others will give in, reluctantly stumbling along paw-burning pavements, panting heavily and craving cool water as you slowly overheat. I cannot for the life of me decide whether these humans are either utterly devoid of any sense, are stuck, mud-like in their routines, or are carrying out a doggie death wish.

Don't feel obliged to greet Tom, Dick or Harry

If you're not an out-going, confident dog, you won't feel comfortable being greeted by every Tom, Dick or Harry human who passes your way. If your human wants you to grow into a happy, balanced dog, they need to understand this and support you.

You'll find some humans think they have a dog-given right to approach and stroke you. To them, anything furry on four-legs, is fair game (though not the flighty, feathered type.) They don't give a second thought to your feelings, or what you may or may not want. They often view themselves as dog whisperers and expect all canines to be cock-a-hoop over their unsolicited approaches.

Even when your mum or dad makes it quite clear to said whisperer that you're a little anxious of strangers and prefer to be left alone, they pay no heed. "Oh, all dogs love me," is the frequent refrain.

Whether you're a fearful rescue, or an anxious pup, the self-satisfying 'dogs-love-me do-gooder' insists on energetically stroking your head or ruffling your ears. I'm surprised more of them don't get bitten, but that's only down to your generous and long-suffering good natures. Should this happen to you, try backing away and hiding safely behind your human. Ideally, it will make Tom, Dick or Harry look and feel a little silly. Only then may these dumb dog-botherers get the message.

Case study: Cariad the Welsh Corgi

Cariad is an active and intelligent chap, but lost the spring in his step due to lack of exercise and stimulation. He told Dr Peter Pointer how much better he felt once his humans realised the issue.

"In my early years Mum and Dad spent quite a bit of time with me. I was well-trained and we had lots of lovely walks together. Mum would also play games with me in the garden. Then Dad began travelling more for work and Mum launched a baking business from home. The smells drifting around the kitchen were delicious, but I noticed I wasn't getting as many walks as I used to. Sometimes I'd only get one quick 20-minute run a day. On other days, if mum had a big order to get out, I didn't get a walk at all.

We didn't play games any more either. I really missed my walks, my games with Mum and my time with Dad. I didn't feel part of the family any more. I'd spend a lot of time curled up in my bed or sniffing around the garden on my own. One day Mum's best friend came to visit. She was a huge dog-lover and very experienced with canines. She helped Mum and Dad with my training and she knew me very well. She noticed immediately how subdued I was. I did get up to greet her but wasn't my usual excited and welcoming self. I then went back to bed. I heard her talking to Mum about me and asking lots of questions about my routine. I pricked up my ears at what she said to Mum next, as it proved a turning point for me. "From what you've told me I think Cariad is depressed. He's a very bright boy and needs plenty of interaction with you. If he has nothing to stimulate him and isn't getting at least one good walk every day, or playing hide and scent games like you used to, his mental health will suffer, which to be honest, I think it already has. He seems very quiet and sad to me. I can see a big difference in him." At that Mum took off her floury apron and knelt down beside me. She cupped her hands around my head. "Oh Cariad, I'm so sorry," she said. I immediately jumped up, wagged my tail and licked her face. This was the first proper mum-time I'd had for weeks. It warmed my heart. "He looks happier already." Mum's friend said. "Come on, let's take him for a walk." From that day on Mum enlisted the help of her friend so I enjoyed daily walks and garden games. In the evening, although she was still icing cakes, Mum set an alarm and would sit with me for 15-minutes. She called it her Cariad time. I soon returned to my happy, adventurous self. I felt part of the family again."

Your sure-pawed route to happiness, is through being well-supported and respected. Consistent boundaries, clear training, appropriate exercise and stimulation are the crucial keys to your mental stability and health. These and these alone, will help you to live a contented life, free from neurosis, obsession, or aggression.

Boredom is often your nemesis. Your clever canine minds don't respond well to having nothing to challenge them. You thrive on daily, off-lead walks, packed with sniffs. Many of you (though not all) enjoy meeting and playing with doggy friends. Others adore agility, fly ball, scent trails, tracking, or mind-boggling games, shared with your human.

Some of you will prefer your own company and your human needs to learn and respect what suits you, as an individual dog. Not all humans are social animals and you are no different.

Humans possess freewill, to make choices in life, but some of you will not be afforded that luxury. This is where you need to show some canine cunning. For instance, if you're picked as a pup from a litter, or seen in a rescue centre kennel, you may need to encourage your chosen human to choose you.

Once you've sussed which human is the one for you (cue your canine intuition) there are means at your doggy disposal to curry favour. It needs a well-timed calm and happy approach, beseeching eye-to-eye contact, a perfect paw here and a loving lick there.

This will help you to touch your would-be human's heart. A similar approach can work well if you're an older, rescue dog. Barking madly and leaping exuberantly at the wire fence is unlikely to endear you to any potential owner. Take it from me, the calm, waggy-tailed, wide-eyed approach always works best.

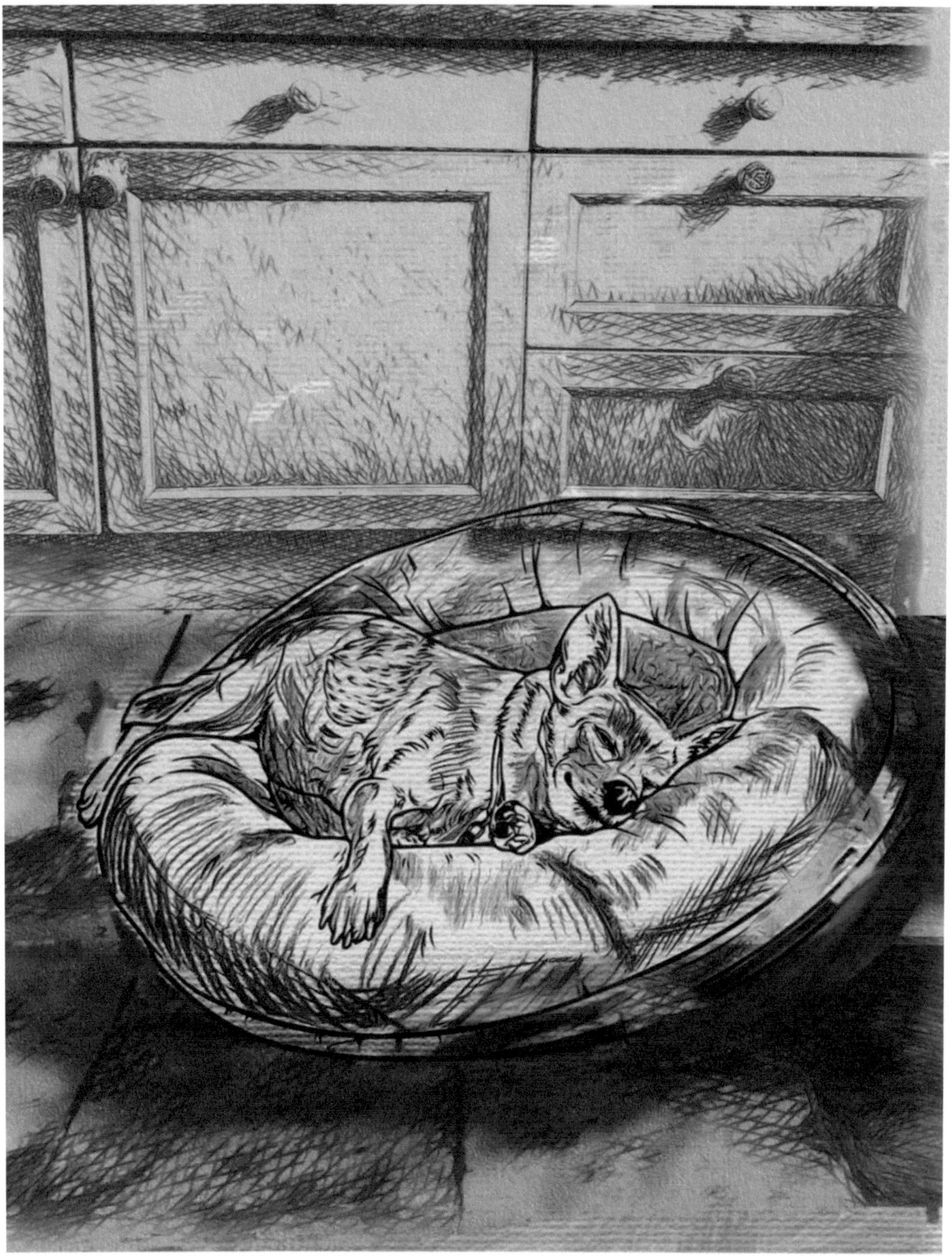

"One of the greatest influences on your ultimate houndy happiness, is the human who shares your life."

For your human to steer you along the right contented canine road, they need to put aside their own desires. They need to consider your needs first - and there are a lot of them. If they focus on your essential doggy dos and don'ts, they'll help you become a content and balanced hound.

Professor Daniel's Bones of Retention:

- **Protect your neck from pulling**
- **Limit limb-use when young**
- **Cheap chews can choke you**
- **Avoid humans who tease you**
- **Doggy socials don't suit everyone**
- **Try calming solutions for stress**
- **There's holistic help for you too**

Chapter 13

You love to love

One thing you may not realise, is that your humongous canine heart is one of the biggest in the universe. Its capacity to love is immense. It has no bottom, no top and no end. In actual fact, it overflows to flooding point with pure love and endless joy. It could be likened to a mountain spring, coming from deep within you, always running fresh and full, brimming over to wash through your lucky humans.

Your love is also unconditional. You love your human whether they have two legs or none, whether their face is stunningly beautiful, or deeply scarred. It matters not a whimper to you, if their eyes don't see you, their ears don't hear you, or their bodies are too big, too small, imperfectly made, or carrying traumatised minds.

You care not a sniff whether they are penniless and live on the streets, or they are wealthy and live in a palace. These differences are only seen and judged by humans. To you, these are superficial matters that won't alter the depth of your love for your human.

Yes, you might have a rather more plush, comfy, padded bed and a large garden and lake to play in if your human is wealthy. But if your human has nothing and lives on the street, you'll still show them the same deep love. They willingly share their food with you, ensure you have a warm blanket to keep out the cold and give you all the love they have.

At the end of the doggy day, it is your human's love for you that is important. You will see and respond to the kindness in their eyes, the gentle touch of their hands and the softness of their voice - for it is these traits that reflect what's in their hearts.

What matters is your human's love for you

You won't be concerned with the size of your bed (though a large comfy one is always welcome). You won't love them any less if you have only one raggedy toy, rather than a whole basketful. Neither will you worry if you don't have the latest fashionable, leather collar, tweed lead, or waterproof, all-weather coat. What does matter, is their love for you and how it's shown.

With humans, there is one big difference between your love and theirs - and it's one of which you need to be well aware. Some humans may love you with conditions, whereas your love comes with absolutely none. You don't love your human because of their big brown eyes, their fluffy coat, their goofy grin, their impeccable and costly pedigree or their latest Crufts certificate. Such a notion is completely alien to you. You love them full-stop. Always and to the end, whether that be your end or theirs, whichever comes first.

It may come as a sobering surprise to you, but sadly, some humans are capable of loving you only with conditions. They probably don't realise this themselves, and you will be so caught up in their lives, you won't either. By conditionally, I mean they can only love you if, for example, you are happy to be carried around in a handbag, or you never trample mud on the carpet, wee in the house, don't bark or whine, or make a nuisance of yourself and always do as you're told. (Though the latter is probably due to a lack of human boundaries or training.)

There are even a few humans whose condition of loving you is that you don't get ill. Whatever your age, you could develop a health condition or have an accident. It may leave you needing drugs for the rest of your life or even surgery. Now these things don't come cheap and some humans don't factor that into the equation when they take you into their homes.

Veterinary treatments come at a cost and some humans simply aren't able or prepared to pay. (Some humans genuinely wouldn't be able to afford the expense and this can result in a heart-breaking scenario for them and for you.) That's one reason why many humans invest in insurance for you. It can help soften the financial blow, should accidents, or illness happen.

Some humans don't show you the same loyalty

I know of older dogs who have given a life-time's love to their human, only to find themselves tied to a rescue centre's railings due to severe arthritis that needs medicating, or left as a pup in a cardboard box at the roadside. Some of the bitches among you, have been quietly cast out after being discovered in pup to a neighbour's rogue male crossbreed.

Case study: Candy the King Charles Spaniel

Candy was used for breeding on a Welsh farm. When the farmer found a big lump on her belly, he took her to a field, let her out and drove off. She tells Dr Peter Pointer what happened next.

"I didn't enjoy my life on the farm. I had two litters of pups a year and spent most of my time in a pen full of straw, in a corrugated iron outbuilding. Sometimes we were allowed out in the yard or field, but not very often. It was exhausting. I never recovered from having one litter before I was mated again for another. I was aware I had this lump growing in my belly and would sometimes lick it from the outside. But I wasn't prepared for being dumped in a field on my own. I had no idea where I was or what to do. I wasn't used to fending for myself and had never spent any length of time in the countryside. I was very disorientated and rather bewildered. It was nice to feel the grass under my paws and hear the birds singing, but I began to feel anxious. I spent the first night hiding under a hedge. It was well past my feeding time and I was very hungry. Luckily, I found a puddle so I could have a drink. A little while later, I picked up the scent of cooking. I followed my nose and found myself in a garden. I count myself very lucky. It was the home of a dog-lover and from that day on, my life changed. Despite having two other dogs, the lady took me in. She tried to trace my owner but of course, that wasn't possible as I was unwanted. She paid for a vet to remove the lump and showered me with love and care. I was bathed, had my nails trimmed, my fur carefully brushed and was given a cosy, warm bed. The vet told her he believed I'd had multiple litters, maybe as many as eight. He put my age at about five-years-old. He was obviously a very

good vet because he was spot on. I never had any more pups and now live the happiest of lives with my new mum."

I know that you would stay by your owner's side and starve to death with them if they weren't able to feed you. But some humans' hearts don't have the same capacity for love, or the ability to show you the same loyalty.

You will love your human come what may - it's your nature. Whatever the ups and downs of their and your lives, you will always be there for them with a snuggle and a lick. Even if you have the misfortune to have a bad being type of human who treats you abysmally, you would still feel it your duty to stay loyal and offer love, even if it's rejected with a cruel kick or a hefty clout.

Case study: Wesley the West Highland Terrier

Wesley lived with his widowed mum in Scotland. They enjoyed many a hike together in the Highlands, but one ended tragically. Recounting the story to Dr Peter Pointer, Wesley's loyalty to his mum never wavered.

"After Dad died, Mum joined a local walking group. I went along too and we had a great time. Mum loved hiking and became more adventurous with her routes. She always took me and we usually went with a friend or two. On this particular day, it was a spur of the moment decision. The sun was shining, so Mum grabbed her stick and backpack and off we drove, just Mum and me. When we arrived, I could tell by the smells it was a new place that we'd not visited before. I felt very excited and was eager to explore. We'd been walking for a couple of hours when I noticed Mum seemed a

bit wobbly and had slowed up. I stayed a bit closer to her. I sensed something wasn't right. As we climbed a shaley path, Mum began gasping for breath and sank to the ground. I knew she was in trouble. We were alone and I was all Mum had. If we'd been nearer to humans, I'd have run for help, but I didn't want to leave Mum up there all alone. Her eyes were closed, so I licked her face a few times and saw a hint of a smile across her mouth. I lay beside her and waited. I hoped someone would come looking for us. It began to get dark and cold. Mum was still asleep. I climbed on top of her chest to keep her warm. I licked her face again, but it was cold and she didn't respond. I tried barking to wake her up, but got no response. I had a feeling she wasn't with me anymore. I wasn't going to leave her and decided to stay with her until someone found us. It was the next morning before we were discovered. I heard voices and barked myself nearly hoarse to alert them. Mum had suffered a heart attack, but died of hypothermia. I really miss Mum and our walks together. I'm glad I was at her side at the end and she knew I was there. The last thing she felt was my lick of love on her face. She didn't die alone."

For those of you who do live with a human with a big heart (though not as big as yours of course), they will most certainly be there for you until your end. For some of you, that may come after a slow decline in your health. It could be the sudden onset of an illness or accident, with no hope of recovery. If you're enduring pain, suffering, and indignity, this is when the size and capacity of your human's heart really comes into its own.

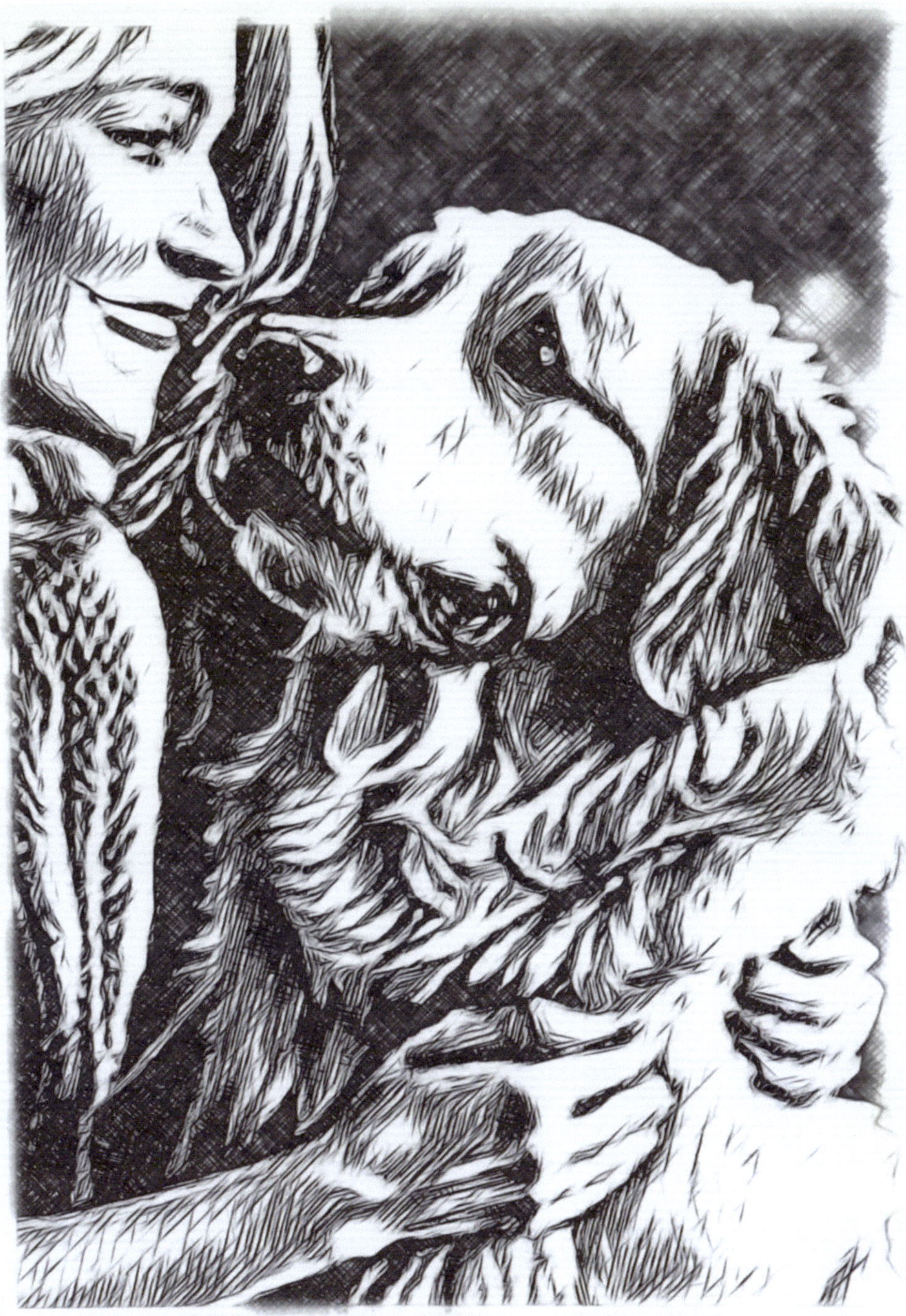

"Your humongous canine heart is one of the biggest in the universe. Its capacity to love is immense."

Those with big hearts will know your time has come. They will make that selfless, agonising decision to let you go, so your suffering is no more. Losing you, will break their hearts but it's the last, love-led, selfless act they can do for you. And believe me they do suffer. Your loving human will be there to cuddle you close and whisper words of comfort in your ear. They will thank you for giving them the purest and deepest love they may ever have the good fortune to experience – yours.

Professor Daniel's Bones of Retention

- **Your heart is humongous**
- **Big-hearted humans are the best**
- **You don't judge**
- **Loyalty is your lifeblood**
- **You love unconditionally**
- **Best buddies are always beside you**
- **Your love is pure**

Chapter 14

Epidogue

I hope you've enjoyed reading this book and are taking something useful from it. My sole aim in putting paws to paper, is to improve the lives of my fellow canines. I hope my Spaniel ramblings raise awareness and understanding among humans, of the finer points of the doggie mind. If this book shines a spotlight on the sensitivity and intelligence of the nation's dogs, I'll be a happy professor. (No, not a bunny.)

I never intended writing a book but was egged on (and I do love a raw egg) by my dear friend and editor, Ruth McDonagh of A Calmer Canine. Ruth works with dogs as a Whole Energy Body Balance (WEBB) Practitioner. (WEBB is a type of massage that releases pain and tension in a dog's neuro-fascia, the connective tissue. It also supports and calms the nervous system).

She convinced me that I had some wise canine words to share, with important messages that needed 'putting out there' as you humans say.

I'd like to extend particular thanks to my esteemed colleague Dr Peter Pointer, PhD (Philosopher of Dogs) who provided the many and varied case studies that are sprinkled throughout the book. These are mostly genuine stories of which he has personal knowledge. We have, of course, changed the names and details of the dogs and their humans for confidentiality and to avoid any paw-pointing. In a couple of instances, Dr Pointer provided fictitious examples of human behaviour based on his professional experience, to demonstrate an issue.

I'm biased of course, but I believe that sharing your life with a dog is a huge privilege, and not to be taken lightly. If you're thinking of becoming a dog-owner, please think long and hard about it. When you welcome a dog, of whatever age, into your home, you are bringing a sentient being into your life.

As I'm at pains to point out throughout this book, a dog feels deeply. It's also extremely knowing; a sensitive soul that experiences joy, sadness, happiness and grief. In fact, I believe the more intelligent and sensitive a dog is, the more likely they are to feel and be affected by human behaviour.

Making a furry addition to your family, is a huge and serious and ongoing commitment. It should be viewed as an unwritten canine contract in which your Terms and Conditions include you providing your canine with love, care, training, exercise, careful socialisation and ongoing stimulation throughout its lifetime. It needs as much time and effort put into its care, as a child – but should not, under any circumstance, be regarded as one.

It's a commitment that also comes with a cost – both financial and emotional. A dog will require significant amounts of money to be spent on it during its 8 – 18-year lifetime, give or take a few years.

The emotional cost – and one that is probably much heavier to bear - is when the time comes to say goodbye. No matter how many dogs you've had, nor how old you are, it gets no easier. For many dog-lovers, losing their pet leaves them as bereft as losing a family member. As far as I'm concerned, there's no shame in that. A dog should be an integral part of your family.

For humans who live alone, a dog becomes a partner of sorts. They talk to it, share much of their time with it and no doubt enjoy lots of walks and adventures together. It's no wonder they're left feeling empty and alone once their four-legged friend is no longer beside them.

If you share your life with a happy hound, there's no question it will bring you years of unbridled pleasure, unquestioned loyalty and unending love.

Even when they've padded quietly out of your life, they will always have a paw-hold on your heart.

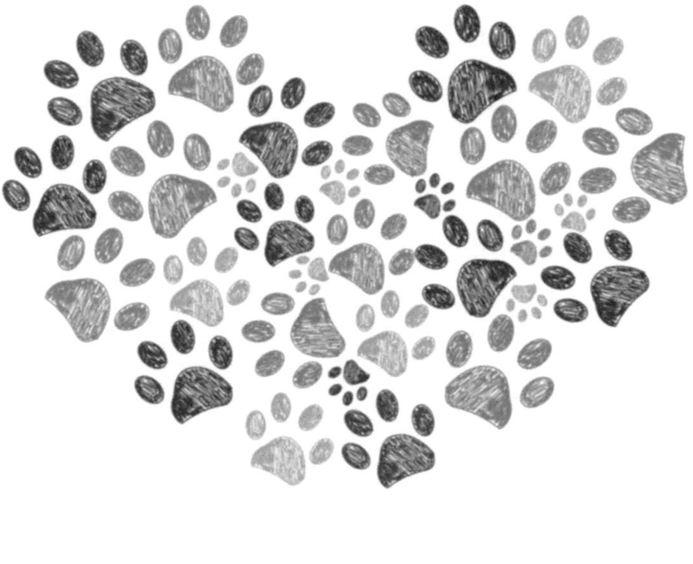

"Even when they've padded quietly out of your life, dogs will always hold a piece of your heart."

Helping your hound: Useful information:

Whole Energy Body Balance
Dog massage with neuro-fascia release and energy therapy:
www.wholeenergybodybalance.com

Whole Energy Body Balance Practitioner Ruth McDonagh, Gloucestershire:
www.a-calmer-canine.co.uk

Whole Energy Body Balance Practitioner and Canine Massage Therapist, Katy Conway, Leicestershire:
www.timeforpooch.co.uk

Whole Energy Body Balance Practitioner Ginny Cunningham, North Wales:
www.calmpetsconwy.co.uk

The Trust Technique
Deepen your bond with your pet:
www.trust-technique.com

Mantrailing UK
Low impact, scent work:
www.mantrailinguk.com

Association of British Veterinary Acupuncturists
www.abva.co.uk

The British Association of Homeopathic Veterinary Surgeons
www.bahvs.net

UK Animal Communicators

Margrit Coates
www.theanimalhealer.com
www.margritcoates.com

Pea Horsley
www.animalthoughts.com

Applied Zoopharmacognosy and Animal Self-Medication

Caroline Ingraham Animals, Botanics, Education

www.carolineingraham.com

www.ingrahamshop.com

Please note: Holistic therapies should not be used as a substitute for veterinary care. Only vets can diagnose illness or injury in animals and prescribe medication. A vet should always be your first port of call if you have concerns over your pet's health.

The details of practitioners and bodies included above are for your reference. It is your responsibility to ensure any holistic therapist you engage, is qualified, insured and a member of a professional body. The author takes no responsibility for services provided by third parties.

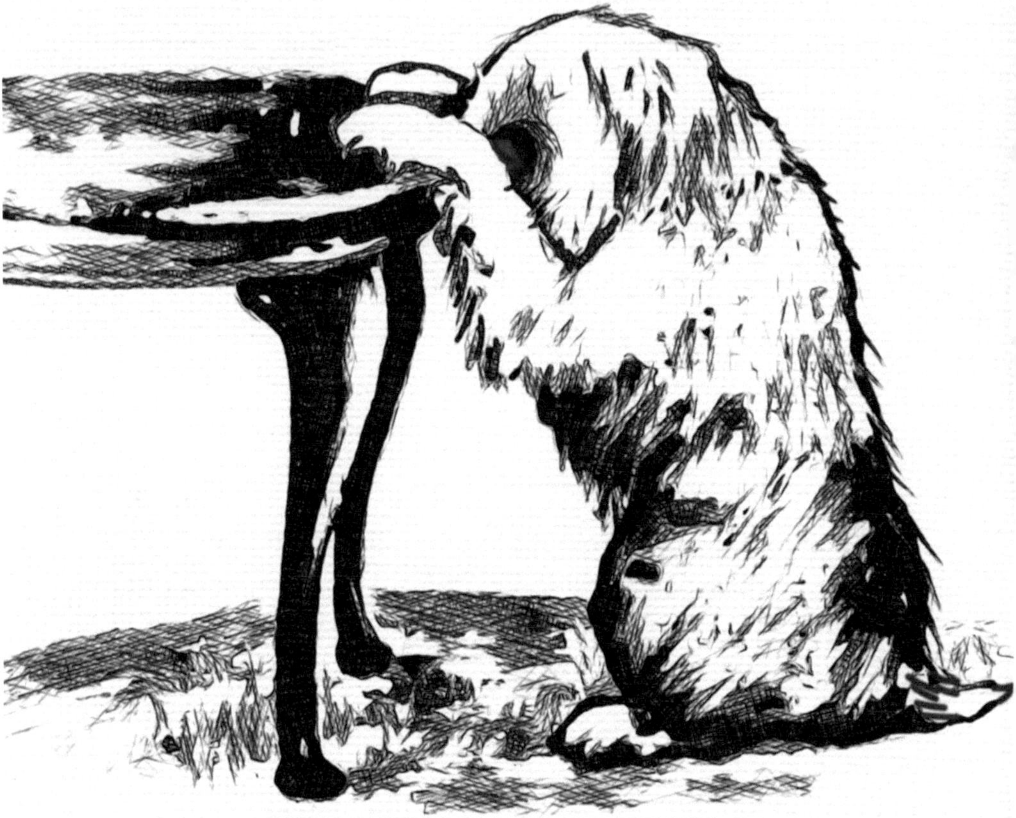

A Little Dog's Prayer

A human who's considerate and kind,
And understands a doggie mind,
Who walks and feeds and loves me each day,
That's all I ask for when I pray.

Author unknown, circa 1950s

Acknowledgements

A big 'Write That Book' thank you goes out to Michael Heppell, one of the UK's top motivational trainers and an international, best-selling author. I took part in his last Write That Book masterclass in November 2022 and it was during the first session the idea for this book emerged. I was so inspired, enthused and motivated by Michael and fellow writers in the group that I carried on writing - and writing and writing!

A special thank you goes to my dear Dad for his unstinting support. I'm extremely grateful to my good friend Sarah Grundy, for her excellent proofreading skills and feedback on all things editorial. Your input and support meant so much. To fellow dog-lover Jane Parry of Happy Hounds, for our endless chats about all things canine and to my Whole Energy Body Balance Practitioner buddy Katy Conway, for her valued input.

I'm indebted to artist Nichola Kingsbury who created the amazing illustrations for this book. She transformed my words into the wonderful characters featured here and brought their emotions to life, patiently making my changes.

To dedicated typesetter Matt Bird, for his marvellous input, advice and layout skills. He held my metaphorical paw throughout the typesetting and design process.

Anyone who has written a book will be familiar with the feeling of overwhelming self-doubt. You question the quality of your words, your ability to write engaging content and whether anyone in their right mind will want to read your book – let alone buy it!

Thank you to all those who have taken an interest in the progress of this book. You won't realise it, but your encouragement helped keep me going.

A heart-felt, heavenly thank you goes out to my dear, late mum, who's been guiding me throughout.

Finally, to all the wonderful dogs who've shared my life so far and to those I've met and continue to work with through A Calmer Canine - you are p-awesome! These sensitive creatures teach me so much and it's a privilege to play a small part in enriching their lives. Dogs are such beautiful souls, whose sentience is often overlooked by us humans. 'They're All Barking', is a tribute to their unstinting love and utter devotion.

About the Editor

Ruth McDonagh spent most of her career as a journalist and freelance copy writer. She grew up in the Cotswolds and for as long as she can remember, has had a deep love for and affinity with dogs. After years of pestering, she was given her first puppy aged 10 and has had at least one, four-legged friend at her side ever since.

Fulfilling her life-long dream of working with dogs, Ruth is now a Whole Energy Body Balance Practitioner, having trained with Dr Edward Bassingthwaite, The Healing Vet.

Through her business A Calmer Canine, she now helps dogs of all shapes, sizes and breeds, who are suffering with a range of emotional and physical issues, and supports their owners. Ruth still lives in the Cotswolds with her rescue Labrador Gem.

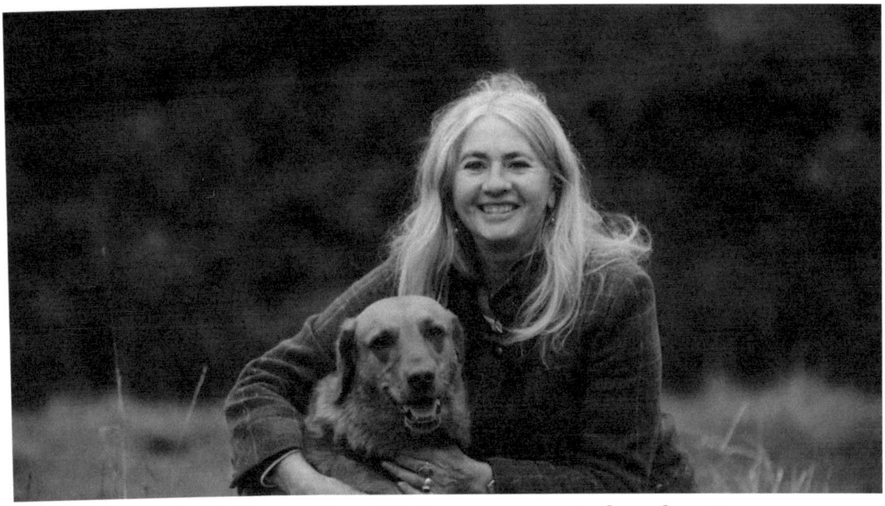

Ruth McDonagh with her rescue Labrador Gem.

Find out more about Ruth's work at
www.a-calmer-canine.co.uk
Connect on Facebook and Instagram.

To buy copies of this book visit **www.professordaniel.co.uk**
To get in touch email **editor@professordaniel.co.uk**